"*Fit for Success* is a great tool to help you become the best you. It makes you think and it offers concrete examples of how you can change the way you approach challenges. I've learned that most situations are not inherently good or bad; they are categorized by how you react to them. *Fit for Success* has helped me to identify when these situations occur and to make conscious decisions about how I respond."

—ANNIE THORISDOTTIR, Two-time Crossfit Games champion

"For seekers of knowledge who want a concise and enjoyable read that covers the spectrum of philosophy and psychology, Nick Shaw provides a book on leadership and holistic living that is both educational and inspiring."

—DANIEL LUNA, retired Navy SEAL and Leadership Coach

"*Fit for Success* is an insightful, practical guide to navigating the real-world situations that so many people face. Nick Shaw has a way of getting to the root of the issue and giving suggestions about how to make lasting changes, not fads. It reads like a letter from a friend, not just another self-help book."

—NITA STRAUSS, professional guitarist

"Success is built on a foundation of deep knowledge. Nick Shaw has done a truly thorough job ravaging hundreds of books on the topic and has pulled together themes that drive long-term success. A truly useful read."

—GREG CONNOLLY, Founder and CEO of Trifecta

"*Fit for Success* is a compelling exploration of the habits and tools that create positive change. Nick draws on his own personal adversity and response, summarizes a wealth of research in an easily digestible manner, and provides real and actionable insights you can put into practice today. *Fit for Success* is easy to read, insightful, and a must-have for anyone on the path of personal or professional betterment."

—MICHAEL SHORETZ, Founder and CEO of Enlightened Ice Cream

"Success cannot be guaranteed, but by applying the simple practices described in this book, you can meaningfully increase your chances of obtaining it. It's not a magic fix, but it's a great start."

—DR. MIKE ISRAETEL, Olympic nutrition consultant, competitive bodybuilder, and PhD in Sport Physiology

"Nick breaks down the nuances of success into an easily digestible, fun-to-read book. His insights can be applied across all areas of life, including my patients trying to lose weight. Anyone trying to achieve success in their life should read this book."

—DR. SPENCER NADOLSKY, Board-Certified Family Physician and Obesity/Lipid Specialist

"This book feels like it was made for 2020—a year full of adversity. Its contents, however, are timeless. I've found my long-term success as a husband, father, businessman and multi-year CrossFit Games Champion through the constant pursuit of behaviors and habits that make me better than I was yesterday. In this book, Nick has skillfully drawn a roadmap for creating and implementing those habits, so you can find success as well."

—RICH FRONING, 8-time CrossFit Games champion

"Nick Shaw is a builder of people and a pioneer in the personal development industry. His passion and knowledge have been an extremely valuable combination helping to accelerate the growth and success of our baseball program. Anyone wanting to maximize their potential or the potential of their team would benefit from Nick Shaw and *Fit for Success*."

—ERIK BAKICH, Head Coach of the University of Michigan baseball team and 2019 NCAA Coach of the Year

"Nick Shaw has a proven record of putting success principles into action. This book promises to be an essential read for anyone who wants to tackle the challenges of business, sport, and life head-on."

—PHIL ANDREWS, CEO of USA Weightlifting

"Those who know Nick Shaw and his company, Renaissance Periodization, will quickly realize this book sticks tightly to his core values of evidence-based practice to help people achieve their full potential. *Fit for Success* combines years of experience gained in the health and fitness industry; extensive business, psychology, and self-help work; and meaningful personal stories into a fun, helpful, and easy-to-read book."

—LORI PLOUTZ-SNYDER, Dean of the University of Michigan's School of Kinesiology

FIT FOR
SUCCESS

FIT FOR
SUCCESS

LESSONS ON ACHIEVEMENT

AND LEADING YOUR BEST LIFE

NICK SHAW

STORY FARM

Published in the United States of America by Story
Farm, Inc.
www.story-farm.com

Library of Congress Cataloging-In-Publication-Data
available upon request.

ISBN 978-0-578-76555-6

Editorial director / Bo Morris
Lead editor / Shaun Tolson
Art director / Jason Farmand
Copy editor / Laura Paquette
Production manager / Tina Dahl

Printed in Canada by Friesens Corporation

First edition, December 2020
10 9 8 7 6 5 4 3 2 1

To my children, Zachary and Emma:
I hope that I can be an example to
you, inspiring you to achieve your own
extraordinary success on whatever path
in life you choose to take.

IT IS MY GOAL to help more than a million people around the world through my company, Renaissance Periodization, and I hope that through this book I am also able to help you. I want to personally thank you for reading it, and I hope that you are able to take a lot from it.

I strongly believe that we have all seen the worst that 2020 has to offer. Because of that, we all have the opportunity to better appreciate the good in the world as we move forward. Remember, every day is a gift. So let's make the most of it and become successful together!

I hope that you will share with me your success stories and the victories that you have taken from this book. You can find me on Instagram: @nick.shaw.rp.

Sincerely,

CONTENTS

PREFACE

—

ON JANUARY 14TH, five days before my son's eighth birthday, I sat in a doctor's office and listened as a nurse advocate relayed the results of a mammogram and a biopsy of a tiny bump that I had found near my right armpit a few months earlier. "There were cancer cells present in the biopsy," she said.

From that moment on, everything changed.

I learned that I had stage-two breast cancer that was "triple negative," meaning it was the most aggressive form of cancer that there is. I elected to have a double mastectomy the following month, but during surgery it was detected that the cancer had spread to two of my lymph nodes, so those were removed as well. Shortly after returning home from the surgery, a complication arose that collapsed half of my lung and sent me back to the hospital for three painful days, during which I was intubated with a chest tube. One month later, I started a sixteen-week round of aggressive chemotherapy, which was followed by five intensive weeks of equally aggressive radiation. To make matters even worse, only one week into my chemotherapy treatments, the coronavirus pandemic reached the United States and forced me to endure those chemotherapy treatments by myself.

During all of that, I had a choice to make. I could ball up in the corner, crying my eyes out every day over the cruel hand I had been dealt and lashing out at everyone for this horrible thing that shouldn't have happened to me. Or I could feel all of those emotions—as anyone would—but then swipe them off my screen and focus on getting better and being positive.

It didn't take me long to choose how I wanted to react. Within days of my diagnosis, I decided I was going to surround myself with positivity—mostly for and because of my kids. I was determined to remain the strong, happy, loving, involved, supportive, and funny mom that they had always known. I also knew from my husband's reading and research that optimism and a positive mindset can play a role in healing and recovery.

In fact, many of the practices of self-improvement that Nick, my husband, had learned over his years of reading and research were applicable to my situation. I began meditating every day, for example. Throughout treatment, I didn't push myself too hard—I gave myself plenty of grace on the days I didn't feel well—but I made sure to get outside every day in the spring to enjoy gardening with my kids. Honestly, those spring blooms got me through some dark days. Ultimately, I focused on the things that I could be grateful for, like savoring meals with my family. I chose happiness and positivity.

I'm not a superstar athlete like many of the contrib-

utors to this book—the people we work with at Renaissance Periodization. But the principles that they follow to
achieve their goals—and the principles that are outlined in
this book—are what helped me to successfully overcome a
serious cancer diagnosis. Not only that, but they are instrumental in my ability to live a happy and successful life
going forward.

Lori Shaw
September 2020

FOREWORD

—

I REMEMBER MEETING Nick Shaw more than 5 years ago, the way that so many people these days do—through social media. I was heavily into the CrossFit world at the time and when I saw RP Strength's before-and-after transformations I thought to myself, *I gotta meet this guy!* Nick and I began corresponding on Instagram and eventually he came out to meet me at my gym in Chelsea. I liked him immediately.

I have been helping people with their diet and exercise plans for as long as I can remember. I've been in the health and fitness industry for more than 25 years. I've worked with overweight people as a trainer on NBC's hit show *The Biggest Loser* for 18 seasons. You could say that I'm completely obsessed with anything related to health and fitness. There really isn't an exercise routine or diet plan that I haven't tried or researched thoroughly. Naturally, I wanted to learn absolutely everything about RP Strength—straight from the man himself. Nick took me on as a client and we began speaking daily.

The teacher had now become the student (and I think Nick would agree that I'm a really good student.) He gave me my plan and we were off! He told me that not only was my body going to change but my performance in the gym would, too.

What I loved about Nick's program was that it wasn't about cutting any major macronutrients. I was so excited that not only could I eat complex carbs, but it was encouraged almost every time I sat down to eat a meal. The key to Nick's program was *balance*. Balance in measuring out all of your macros: protein, fat, and carbs, and on top of that adding your fresh leafy greens and veggies.

I've always wanted to train smart and Nick assured me that the fuel that I would be getting from my food would work for me in the gym and *boy did it!* I started performing much better and felt the fittest I had been in years. Everyone I regularly worked out with noticed the difference. I felt like I found a secret treasure map and at the "X" there was box filled with rice, pasta & bread! For me, when I depleted my body of carbs, I felt like a fish swimming upstream and when I began to give my body what it needed, it gave me the results I wanted. It was a match made in heaven.

Fast forward a couple of years and I'm working out in the same gym where I first met Nick, unaware that my life was about to change forever. It was Sunday, February 12, 2017, a day that I have no memory of whatsoever. I don't remember getting up that morning to take my dog for a walk or walking to the gym for my workout with friends. I was told that I had complained of feeling dizzy, and in the middle of the workout I just went to the ground. I was having a "widow-maker" heart attack. And not only that, but I also went into cardiac arrest.

They call it a widow-maker for a reason. Only about 10 percent of people survive. If it wasn't for the fast action of the staff calling 911, grabbing the AED, and finding a doctor that just happened to be there that day for an event, I would not be writing this foreword right now. Two days later, I woke up in the hospital after being put into a medically induced coma. When I was told what had happened, I couldn't believe it. To top it off, I was also experiencing short term memory loss, like Dory in *Finding Nemo*. I would be told why I was in the hospital, I would get super emotional, and then a few minutes later I would have to ask again what happened and why I was in the hospital. It was a very surreal time, and I can honestly say it was the hardest time of my life.

When I was finally discharged from the hospital a week later, I was just trying to figure out what my "new normal" was going to be. I had to change everything about the way that I worked out and the way that I was supposed to eat. I'm not a person that adapts to change very well so it was definitely challenging. I went from Olympic-style weightlifting and pushing my body to extremes in the gym to just walking at 2.5 mph on a treadmill in cardiac rehab and riding a recumbent bicycle. For several months, the only thing I was allowed to do outside of rehab was walk. At first I could only get around the block before I would get winded and have to come back home. Time and patience increased my walking distance, and by following the strict instructions from my doctors, I started to feel physically stronger.

Everything about my life had to change and that included my diet. I made the decision to reach back out to Nick and to sit down with him to figure out a plan that was going to be right for me and be on par with what my doctors wanted me to do. I had a history with Nick and I trusted him completely. I knew I was in good hands. Nick gave me a roadmap to my new way of eating. I needed balance now more than ever, and when I talked to Nick about my new dietary restrictions, he had all the answers. He also hooked me up with a trainer to make sure I was comfortable in the gym again.

I no longer felt like I needed to leave it all out on the gym floor when I worked out. I just wanted to feel confident again and ultimately, just feel good. Nick heard me and adapted to what I needed. For that, I will always have nothing but love and respect for him. This man is the real deal. Not only is he knowledgeable about eating sensibly and working out effectively, he really does care. He's the perfect balance of caring, leadership, and information. When you hear what he has to say, you just want to do it because you know that you are in very good hands.

I believe in Nick and the fundamentals of what he teaches. To make real changes you have to have both discipline and a positive mindset, which are two of the pillars in his program. Not surprisingly, they are also two of the pillars in Nick's roadmap to success, which is the focus of this book. Just like he does through his fitness company, Renaissance Periodization, Nick has created a program in this book that focuses on the behaviors and the habits that can lead to success.

Nick Shaw has been a blessing in my life, and I know that through this book he can be that same blessing for you.

Bob Harper
September, 2020

INTRODUCTION

———

JANUARY 14, 2020. It's a date that I will never forget. For the first eight hours, the day felt like a normal Tuesday. I helped my wife, Lori, get our seven-year-old son and five-year-old daughter ready for school, then I drove them to the town's elementary school. After a couple of hours spent catching up on work emails, paying bills, and checking in with various Renaissance Periodization team members all over the country, I went to the gym to get a workout in for myself.

Lori had a doctor's appointment at 1:30 that afternoon, but because our kids needed to be picked up at school around 2:00, we couldn't both go to the appointment. Lori left to go see her doctor and I stayed home to pick up the kids an hour or so later. Just as I was getting ready to hop in the car, my phone rang. It was Lori. When I answered, I could immediately tell that something was wrong. She was crying.

That's when I learned that my wife had breast cancer.

This can't be right, I kept thinking as I listened to my wife share this horrible news while I drove to the elementary school. *This has to be wrong. Lori is in great shape—she's young and she's healthy.* I realize now that this thought process is the default mode that people immediately shift into when they're given this type of diagnosis. We didn't have enough information yet. We didn't know how bad it was or what stage Lori was in. All we knew was that she had cancer.

No one ever expects to get bad news like that. I was in shock.

Up until then I had lived a life entirely devoid of tragedy. Thankfully, both of my parents were still alive and the only deaths in the family—my maternal grandmother and paternal grandfather—had occurred before I was born. For thirty-two years I lived a life having never experienced truly devastating news. This diagnosis changed all of that.

Three and a half weeks later, Lori had surgery to remove the tumor. The procedure was a success, but she still faced almost four months of chemotherapy, and then radiation treatments after that. Shortly after the surgery, a pandemic caused by the outbreak of Covid-19 began to spread across much of the world. By the end of February, that pandemic had reached the United States and our own, personal world was thrust into chaos.

I HAD ONLY TAKEN LORI to one chemotherapy appointment, her first, when shelter-in-place orders were issued across much of the country. That meant I would have to balance working at home with the homeschooling of our two kids and also help my wife to manage her chemotherapy treatments, only now she would have to drive herself to the cancer center. On top of all that, there was the stress of knowing that the economy was in potential turmoil. As the unemployment rate spiked and gyms closed, I was worried about losing customers. I was also worried about the forty-five members of the Renaissance Periodization team. I didn't want my employees or coaches to suffer, and I certainly didn't want to lay anyone off. But I also didn't know what to prepare for. It felt like the world was ending.

At that moment, it would've been easy for me to play the victim card. Fortunately, I was well prepared to take on these challenges. In the fall of 2018, a hernia surgery derailed my strength training regimen. After the surgery I could only walk initially, so I began listening to audio books while I walked around the neighborhood. It started with *Rich Dad, Poor Dad*—I wanted to make sure I was doing everything right for my family's finances and to improve my business—but it quickly snowballed from there. I read as many books as I could get my hands on, listening to audiobooks or podcasts whenever I was in the car. Before long, I was only reading or listening to self-improvement books. Over the course of a few months, I began to spot trends in all of the various principles taught in those self-improvement books, and I soon discovered how they were all interrelated.

As Lori battled breast cancer and the world went haywire thanks to a global pandemic, I knew I couldn't be a passive victim in these circumstances. In doing so, I would relinquish the power that I had to impact our future. This was the moment when I was forced to put into action all the lessons that I had learned from my reading. We still had a long, hard road ahead of us, and it was time to put my hypothesis to the test.

A person's mindset is one of the key pillars of success. In fact, there are seven main habits to success, and a strong work ethic lays the foundation. That is where everything starts and where change can begin; however—as I learned—without the right mindset, it's impossible for anyone to be successful, whether in sports, business, or battling cancer.

I realize that I have been incredibly fortunate up to this point in my life. I was raised the right way by two incredibly hardworking parents, I have a great family, and I've built a successful business. Through my own experiences and the information that I've gathered from extensive reading on the subject of self-improvement, I have created a roadmap to success. It's an approach to successful living that has worked for me, and it's supported by the experiences and habits of many others, all of which are shared in this book.

As a global pandemic continues to impact the world, it's easy to feel overwhelmed. It's also easy to feel powerless. But if you are equipped with the right knowledge, you can successfully overcome any obstacles in your way.

THE HABITS
OF SUCCESS

—

AT RENAISSANCE PERIODIZATION (RP), my team and I have published numerous diet and strength training books that address the hierarchical nature of the factors that lead to success. We view those hierarchies like a pyramid made up of different levels. The most fundamental factors form the base of the pyramid, while other necessary aspects tied to those fundamentals make up the middle sections. The least impactful factors—the ones that aren't critical to general success but are crucial to obtain the best possible results—form the top of the pyramid.

In much the same way, the habits of success that are featured in this book form a similar hierarchy. Some are foundational: without them, success simply isn't possible. Others are core pieces to maximize success, while some take the form of success-enhancers. Interestingly, each one builds off of the more significant habit that precedes it.

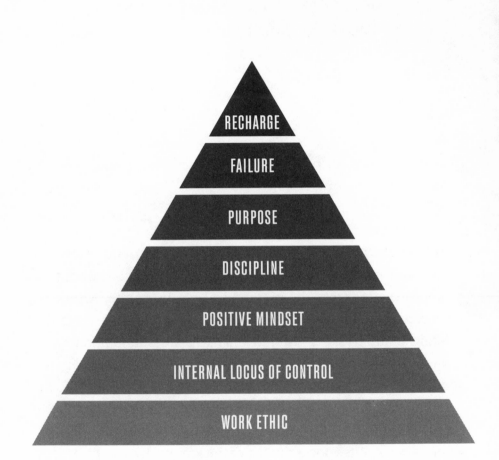

Let's take a closer look at the seven key habits to success that we'll explore in greater detail in the chapters ahead, starting with the most significant components and working our way up the pyramid:

1. WORK ETHIC
By definition, this is the most foundational habit for success in any venture. A strong work ethic is critical, since success itself is only possible through the application of hard work.

2. INTERNAL LOCUS OF CONTROL
This is the belief that individuals—not external forces— have control over the outcomes of the events in their lives. Hard work is necessary for success, and it's imperative to recognize that you are the one tasked with doing that work. It's also important to recognize what you can and cannot change. That understanding will allow you to focus your hard work on the right initiatives.

3. POSITIVE MINDSET
You may be a hard worker with an exceptional locus of control, but it's still possible that you may find yourself feeling overwhelmed. You may even become pessimistic about your limited abilities and how much you think you can change. For those reasons, it's important that you remain positive. An optimistic mindset actually increases your chances of success.

4. DISCIPLINE

It's not always going to be smooth sailing. Sometimes, you will have to really dig in to get things done, and that requires discipline.

5. PURPOSE

Even with a positive mindset, a sharp locus of control, a strong work ethic, and plenty of discipline, things can derail you. In particular, you may find yourself getting off track and focusing on less important projects. Knowing your purpose will help you to target your productivity, making sure that you're not simply doing things, but that you're doing the right things. If, at some point during the process, you ask, "What am I grinding for?" your purpose will provide the answer. It will also help you to stay disciplined and to keep going.

6. FAILURE

You can be as disciplined as humanly possible, with a strong work ethic, a positive mindset, and a resolute focus on your purpose, yet there will be times when you will still fail. It's just going to happen from time to time, but how you choose to deal with it can determine how successful you ultimately become.

7. RECHARGE

All of this seems a bit draining, doesn't it? The truth is, it can be. Even the most highly disciplined and driven folks can burn out. That is why it's important to recharge. You can do this through exercise and nutrition, through personal growth, and through meditation and self-reflection.

Now that you understand how the pyramid is structured, let's examine each habit individually, including how you put them into practice.

CHAPTER 1

WORK ETHIC

" —
"Be humble. Be hungry. And always
be the hardest worker in the room."

—DWAYNE JOHNSON

THE NOTION OF WORKING HARD or being a hard worker is such a commonly extolled virtue that saying as much borders on banality. "Of course hard work is required!" people will say, rolling their eyes. And they have a point: hard work is so universally espoused as the key to success that it's easy to assume it is the only requisite ingredient.

However, hard work is often, dare I say, *overrated*. Don't get me wrong, working hard is important, especially if you want to be successful. But the extent of how hard you work isn't always commensurate with the amount of success you ultimately achieve. A construction worker who diligently applies himself and works hard every day is likely to earn a promotion. In that example, the level of success reflects the level of hard work that was applied. But is it also true that the most successful artists are the ones who also work the hardest? Almost certainly not. In fact, the best artists— in most cases—are the sculptors or painters who have the greatest amount of natural talent.

THE RELATIONSHIP BETWEEN WORK AND SUCCESS

Hard work alone will not guarantee you success. But it plays two influential roles in determining the amount of success that you ultimately achieve. As you already know, success is the byproduct of several different factors; any success that you achieve as a result of those other factors is magnified by the amount of effort that you put in. If you're talented, you'll be more successful the harder you work. If you get lucky, hard work will capitalize on that luck and net even greater results. If you have a strong support network, then the harder you work, the more you can utilize that network to accomplish great things.

That's the role that hard work plays as a supporting player. But supporting players rarely win MVP awards and hard work—as you'll recall—forms the base of our pyramid. That means it's not just a supporting player, it's also your team's superstar. That brings us to the more impactful role that hard work plays.

Simply put, hard work is the only thing that actually *creates* success. A brilliant inventor might have hundreds of amazing ideas, but if he or she is too lazy to write them down, to expand on them, and to do the legwork to develop them, then that inventor will achieve zero success. The most talented baseball pitchers don't strike out batters or win games just because they have talent. They still have to throw the ball.

In a direct sense, work *causes* success. And in some cases, the minimum amount of work that is required for success can be quite high. Creating a vaccine requires scientists to spend hundreds, if not thousands, of hours working diligently in their laboratories. Computer programmers must write hundreds of thousands of lines of code if they want to create an effective computer program. And Olympic weightlifters must train for thousands of hours if they want any chance to represent their countries and to compete on the world's grandest stage.

Failing to meet these minimum thresholds of effort doesn't lead to less success, but no success at all. Programmers who don't finish writing the necessary lines of code will develop not a less functional program, but one that does nothing useful whatsoever. And chemists who don't log all the necessary hours of research in the bio lab won't create a less-effective vaccine. They simply won't create a vaccine. The hard truth of the matter is this: if you want to be successful in the modern world, you have to work long and hard just to have a chance at it.

Hard work is unique. Think of it like the engine of a satellite-launching rocket. It doesn't matter how advanced the rocket's navigation system is or how amazing the satellite payload might be if the engine thrust to take it into space is missing. Of course, engine thrust by itself won't produce a successful launch. But without the thrust from a good engine, nothing at all can happen. Hard work is your engine thrust—and it matters a great deal how willing you are to do that work.

STRENGTHENING YOUR DESIRE TO WORK

"I was brought up to believe that I could do anything I wanted to if I was willing to put in the work," says Annie Thorisdottir, a two-time CrossFit Games champion. "I have always poured my heart into everything I have done. Do it at 100 percent effort or not at all."

In simple terms, successful people have three related abilities in great abundance—the ability to work hard, the desire to do it, and the commitment to follow through on it. In many respects, the ability to do the work is dependent on talent or skill. A farmer might need to load 100-pound jugs of water onto a truck bed, for example, but if he cannot lift one-hundred pounds, he won't be successful because he can't do the work that is required. Similarly, a musician who lacks the talent to compose won't be able to create anything noteworthy of his or her own.

Ability is critical, but desire is the big magnifier. Take the example of the farmer. Even if he is capable of lifting 100-pound jugs of water, he may have no desire to do it. Therefore, true work ethic requires not just the ability to do the work, but the desire to do it and the commitment to follow through. Ability and desire are important factors, but you cannot overlook being committed to the work. You can have all the ability and desire in the world, but you must be capable of following through and committing to that work if you want to be successful.

Fortunately, there are ways to improve your work ethic. In fact, there are ways to strengthen all three factors of it: your ability, your desire, and your commitment. You can improve your ability to do the work by learning—if the work is cerebral in nature—as well as through practice. The old adage that practice makes perfect may or may not be true, but practice definitely improves overall ability. It can also enhance your desire to do the work. Past success also plays a role in enhancing desire, as does meditation on the relationship between work and success. A person's desire to work hard acts like a volume knob on their success. The more they turn up their desire, the greater their success (or potential success) becomes. In other words, the stronger your desire for success, the more you'll want to do the work that is needed to achieve it. Finally, you can enhance your commitment to follow through on tasks in a number of ways, the simplest of which is a daily to-do list. By making a list of must-do tasks every morning (or the night before), you can hold yourself accountable to getting done what needs to get done. Tracking your commitment becomes as easy as checking a box, and by selecting realistic (but still challenging) daily tasks, you can build a habit of completing projects that will keep you on the path to success.

At its core, success is achieved through difficult tasks that are consistently completed. Therein lies the significance of a strong work ethic. No amount of motivational tricks, mindfulness practices, or self-care will ever *create* anything. Only work does that. Famous authors are successful—and by extension, famous—because they put in the work to write the books for which they are well known. If you yearn for success, you must be ready to work, eager to work hard, and to see that work through to its completion. That's the key to every success story.

Just working hard, however, will not lead to success. In fact, incredibly talented people can often find themselves overwhelmed by the amount of work that they assume must be done to achieve that success. By failing to focus their work on the specific tasks that matter—instead toiling over the many tasks that matter very little (or don't matter at all)—those incredibly hardworking people can wind up unsuccessful.

To avoid making those mistakes, you'll need to cultivate an internal locus of control.

PUTTING IT INTO PRACTICE

Create and use a daily to-do list: Making a to-do list for each day prioritizes your most important tasks and holds you accountable, which ensures that those tasks are completed. Make sure that you're including tasks that are actually accomplishable that day. These daily to-do lists provide you with incremental successes each day, which create positive momentum to keep you going.

—

CHAPTER 2

INTERNAL LOCUS OF CONTROL

" —
You have power over your mind — not outside events. Realize this, and you will find strength."

—MARCUS AURELIUS

DURING WORLD WAR I, soldiers lived for long periods of time in the trenches, constantly under attack and always fearful of artillery strikes. Two decades later, many soldiers experienced similar psychological conditions during beach invasions in the South Pacific throughout World War II. In both cases, soldiers were at the mercy of those artillery strikes; they had no control over the outcome of those offenses. Their only option was to duck and cover, hoping that nothing happened to them. This style of warfare wreaked havoc on soldiers' psyches.

You might be asking, what does artillery shelling have to do with this book? The answer lies in an individual's ability to control his or her outcome.

Internal locus of control is the degree to which people believe that they, rather than external forces, have control over the outcomes of the events that make up their lives. Soldiers on the offensive, who are assaulting an enemy position, will have more control over their outcomes due to a number of factors, including the size of their platoon and the route that they take to attack their enemies. Those soldiers have an internal locus of control, whereas those who are under a siege of steady artillery do not. The soldiers who are taking cover in the trenches are simply hoping that they'll be lucky and the shrapnel from the blast won't injure or kill them.

Here's a more relatable example. Imagine you are on a diet to lose weight, and you have to take a business trip. Many external factors will pop up during that trip that could derail you. Your flights could be delayed, or colleagues could bring doughnuts into the office. You can't control the timing of your flights or the actions of other coworkers, but you can be prepared by having healthy snack options with you. By taking back the power to make the best of the situation that you are dealt, you are giving yourself an internal locus of control.

When Lori and I learned of her breast cancer diagnosis, Zionna Hanson, the CEO of Barbells for Boobs, offered some helpful advice. Focus on the things you can control, she told us. Don't spend time focusing on the cancer itself—that won't improve anything. You have to shift your focus and your mindset onto the things you have power over. You cannot control your diagnosis, but you can change your mindset, your attitude, and your habits to make sure you kick cancer's ass and get started on the proper road to recovery. In other words, there is always a lot of work to do, but knowing where and how to focus your efforts is crucial.

Just how important is a strong internal locus of control? In his book *Choice or Chance: Understanding Your Locus of Control and Why It Matters*, Stephen Nowicki shares decades of research on the subject and reveals that people who think and believe that they have control over the outcomes of their lives suffer from fewer behavioral problems in school; live longer, healthier lives; are in better control of their finances; and tend to be happier and more satisfied.

STOIC PHILOSOPHY

Marcus Aurelius is widely regarded as one of the top stoic philosophers of ancient Rome. Stoic philosophy draws largely upon the idea of self-control. Aurelius reasoned that regardless of your circumstances or how bad an external event might be or seem, *you* have the ultimate ability to control how you respond to it.

This idea, although ancient in its origin, helps to explain why cognitive behavioral therapy (CBT) has recently become such a well supported mode of therapy. The main premise of CBT is to challenge the cognitive distortions that arise in the mind. If you have a day when you slip up on your diet, for example, you might initially think that you're doomed. That thought can spiral into other negative thoughts, and before long you might be thinking that you're destined to fail at everything. Someone who is conditioned by CBT, however, would think of examples that disprove that generalization. Challenging your own thoughts takes practice, but it can be an effective tool in shaping how you respond to any situation.

The idea is similar to the first habit that Stephen Covey identifies in his best-selling book *The 7 Habits of Highly Effective People*, which emphasizes the importance of being proactive. An individual who is proactive rather than reactive takes a position of power. No matter the circumstances, they can shape how they feel about something. Covey points to Viktor Frankl—who survived being a prisoner in a World War II concentration camp—as the perfect example.

Despite being subjected to terrible conditions and losing his family, Frankl never relinquished control. He focused on the belief that he was meant to survive, that his purpose was to write powerful works like *Man's Search for Meaning*, which could help many more people in the future. That ultimate purpose allowed him to overcome traumatizing obstacles. "Everything can be taken from a man but one thing," he later wrote in *Man's Search for Meaning*, "the last of the human freedoms—to choose one's attitude in any given set of circumstances, to choose one's own way."

FLOW

Can our mindset assert that much control over our lives? Mihaly Csikszentmihalyi, in his book *Flow: The Psychology of Optimal Experience*, asserts that it can. Csikszentmihalyi tells a story about another prisoner of war, Major James Nesmeth. According to Csikszentmihalyi, Nesmeth was taken prisoner during the Vietnam War. Despite being detained in terrible living conditions, Nesmeth shifted his focus to the elements that he could control. Every day he visualized playing eighteen holes of golf. When he was finally released, after years of confinement, Nesmeth returned to the golf course and, despite not having swung a club in years and also being severely malnourished, he played better than he ever had.

To be in a state of flow that produces extreme happiness or enjoyment, Csikszentmihalyi suggests that we must first be in control of our consciousness. We need to choose the outcomes that we wish to seek out. In doing so, we will set specific goals to accomplish and challenges that must be met, which will push us past what we thought possible.

As we do this, we get so caught up in the process that we lose our worries about all external factors. Our sole focus becomes the task or goal at hand as we pursue it. This is how the best professional athletes can perform at such high levels, even when hundreds of thousands of fans are cheering and watching them perform. These athletes are in complete control, but in that moment that control is effortless. That is being in a state of flow.

"The best moments in our lives are not the passive, receptive, relaxing times," Csikszentmihalyi writes. "The best moments usually occur if a person's body or mind is stretched to its limits in a voluntary effort to accomplish something difficult and worthwhile."

To achieve true happiness, we must have a say over what paths we pursue. This idea of flow crosses over into multiple areas, too; the pursuit doesn't necessarily need to be highly physical. For example, while writing this book, I experienced my own state of flow. Many times I would find myself in a zone where I'd be scribbling down notes, interlocking different ideas, and exploring how they all tied together. This book was a challenge that I chose to take on, and in doing so I was able to dive in and push my own limits.

In his book *Flourish: A Visionary New Understanding of Happiness and Well-being*, Martin Seligman identifies the factors that determine a person's general well-being and incorporates state of flow, though he doesn't use those exact words. In his earlier attempts to uncover the source of happiness, Seligman placed most of the significance on positive emotion, but in *Flourish* he expanded on that study, creating the acronym PERMA (Positive Emotion, Engagement, Relationships, Meaning, and Achievement). Positive emotion still plays a pivotal role, but Seligman also alludes to being in a state of flow through the inclusion of "meaning" and "achievement." Remember, to achieve a flow state you must have goals to pursue (meaning) and you must ultimately accomplish them (achievement). In that way, a state of flow not only influences a person's overall well-being, it also plays a role in determining a person's level of success.

AUTONOMY

Having an internal locus of control is important to success—but relinquishing some of that control to coworkers or subordinates is also a necessary step. To do so, you must trust the power of autonomy. When giving your colleagues autonomy, you present them with an overall goal and let them decide which course of action is best to take. You trust that they have the talents and abilities to accomplish the task at hand. You don't micromanage. This takes time, so you must either train your employees effectively from the start or you must hire smart and qualified people who know more than you do. That is the only way you can develop complete trust in them and their capabilities.

Those with a massive work ethic can struggle with relinquishing control, but by not providing the people that you work with (and those who work for you) autonomy, you can negatively impact your own success. I learned that lesson the hard way . . . more than once! My first introduction to the importance of autonomy came during a summer internship when I was in college. We students were given an opportunity to run our own businesses, and for this internship that business took the form of a painting company. Rather than acting as the owner of the business and hiring a crew to tackle the physical work, I hired a group of my friends—my first mistake—and then worked alongside them as a painter (mistake number two). I spent more time micromanaging the other painters than I did working to improve the business, bringing in more projects, and growing the company.

When I launched Renaissance Periodization several years later, I ended up making a similar mistake at the onset. I adopted the mindset that if things were going to get done, I would have to do them myself. I got so bogged down replying to emails and answering client comments and concerns—all these customer service tasks—that I ran out of time during the day to address the company's marketing and social media campaigns, which were necessary if Renaissance Periodization was to scale up its business. Only when I got out of my own way and hired people to handle those customer service tasks did the business take off. Today, because all of my staff members work remotely, the people that I've hired have a high level of autonomy. And I've learned that when I stay out of the way and let those people do their jobs, it's a win-win.

Daniel Pink addresses the main components of success in *Drive: The Surprising Truth about What Motivates Us*. As he asserts, we all want to have a say and to be in control of where we go and what we do. Offering autonomy gives this feeling of freedom back to your colleagues and teammates and, in doing so, you make sure that everyone moves forward with a heightened internal locus of control. According to Pink, this often produces a more intrinsic motivation, which leads to better (or more) success. Simply put, those individuals will be better aligned with one another and on the same page, even if they take different routes to accomplish the same collective goal.

Intrinsic motivation is key to success because it's literally what keeps people going. External motivations like money or material possessions are nice, but they have a shorter period of effectiveness. Intrinsic motivation, Pink argues, is more sustaining. Paying a child to do household chores, for example, may seem like a great idea, but it will only incentivize them in the short term. They won't gain a sense of satisfaction by completing the task or learning how to master a new skill, and they won't be motivated to complete those chores in the future if pay isn't involved.

Charles Duhigg outlines just how much influence autonomy can have on a company's success in his book *The Power of Habit: Why We Do What We Do in Life and Business*. Duhigg spotlights a manufacturing plant in Ohio that allowed its employees to design and choose their own uniforms. It also provided them with some authority over their shifts. According to Duhigg, those employees' productivity rate increased by 20 percent. "Giving employees a sense of control," he wrote, "improved how much self-discipline they brought to their jobs."

OWNERSHIP

As you now understand, developing an internal locus of control shifts the ownership of any outcome back to you. This pertains to positive outcomes as well as negative ones. If a business deal goes bad, for example, you—as the owner of the company—must accept the blame for it, even if somebody else at your business was ultimately responsible. If you're in a leadership position, you oversaw that employee's training, so it all comes back to you. That is ownership. But owning any issue that arises is also empowering because it means you will also own the solution to those problems. Having ownership of things that go wrong gives you the power to make corrections. Even that contributes to your internal locus of control.

Studies about how people eat have revealed the influence that external forces can have on us if we are not careful. They've also shown how an internal locus of control is paramount to success when dieting. In an experiment detailed in the book *Willpower: Rediscovering the Greatest Human Strength*, two sets of restaurant patrons ordered chicken wings, but waiters constantly cleared the tables of any scraps while the patrons in one of the groups were eating. The other group ate as the remnants of their finished wings remained in sight on the table. Perhaps not surprisingly, the group that had no visible evidence to show them how many they had eaten inevitably overate.

Now's a good place to address social media, since it can be a dangerous reality as far as your locus of control is concerned. Too often, people will compare themselves to others on social media, going so far as to evaluate their own success and happiness by what they see via other people's posts. In doing so, they are relinquishing their own internal locus of control. It's important to acknowledge that social media acts like a highlight reel. By and large, it only offers people a glimpse at the positive aspects of someone's life. Most people do not post their struggles, failures, or regrets. Remember, you have the power to choose how you respond to any external stimulus. You can choose to be jealous or angry about what you see on social media, or you can choose to not let it bother you. Even better, you can use it as fuel for your own success.

You might think that you won't be influenced by other people's circumstances or the details of their lives versus your own, but consider this: in 1997 the *Quarterly Journal of Economics* published the results of a survey where 80 percent of the people polled said that they would rather make $34,000 per year (when the average salary was $30,000) than $36,000 per year (when the average salary was $40,000). Think about that. The vast majority of people preferred to make $2,000 less per year only because that particular salary compared more favorably to the average.

Successful people tend not to give away their control and power to others. They are not concerned with keeping up a certain look or appearance, especially when that money can be better spent on themselves or reinvesting in their own success. Before you go out and buy that fancy car or take that exotic trip, ask yourself why you are really doing it. Consider your own ego and then make the best choice for yourself in the long run, not just for immediate gratification. It takes a lot of discipline to do that, but if you start training your mind to think that way, you'll find it easier as time goes by.

You may believe that you won't fall victim to this, but think about the trips you take and the types of gifts you buy for your family and friends. Are you spending too much just because of the new norms that social media has created? According to *Parenting* magazine, 76 percent of parents spoil their kids to avoid feeling guilty. "Mentally strong people," Amy Morin wrote, "don't waste energy on things they can't control." Remember that.

LUCK

Is a strong work ethic and an internal locus of control all we need? Could there be any external factors at work? The answer is decidedly yes. In 1926, George S. Clason wrote as much in *The Richest Man in Babylon*, a book of financial advice that he founded on the teachings of many 4,000-year-old parables. "Men of action," he wrote, "are favored by the Goddess of good luck."

Luck does play a factor, but believe it or not, you can even have some control over how lucky you might end up being. First, you need to be, as Clason surmises, a person of action. If you never take a chance and you never get going, you'll never be in a position to benefit from luck. You must first have the work ethic to produce what is necessary, as well as the accountability over your own actions to steer your efforts in the right direction. Once that action is put into place, your luck increases. Think of playing the lottery. It's the ultimate game of luck, but you can't win anything if you don't first buy a ticket.

That being said, there is a time and place for luck to factor in. Malcolm Gladwell addresses this in his book *Outliers*. Bill Gates, Steve Jobs, and Scott McNealy were all born within a few years of each other, and each stumbled upon computing technology in the industry's early years. Gladwell suggests that the timing represents their good luck. But simply being born between 1954 and 1956 didn't give those three entrepreneurs an immense advantage. They still had to put in the work to create their business empires. They just benefited from a little bit of luck that put them in the right place at the right time to take advantage of the opportunity.

Of course, there are occasional times in business when

luck in its truest sense can make a difference. In his book *The Success Equation: Untangling Skill and Luck in Business, Sports, and Investing*, Michael. J. Mauboussin shares a story about a job interview that he had early in his career. As Mauboussin reveals, one of the company's managers connected with him over their shared love of the same Washington, D.C., football team. That gave Mauboussin an advantage over the other candidates—at least in the eyes of that particular manager. If Mauboussin gets the job because of his allegiance to a particular football team, suddenly he is thrust into a business environment surrounded by influential colleagues and better resources. That opportunity becomes a catalyst for future opportunities that the other candidates might never receive. So, by projecting the rest of Mauboussin's career, you can see how one element of luck at the start can set him on a different, more successful path than other equally qualified candidates who were interviewing for that same job.

THE RISKS OF HAVING TOO MUCH CONTROL

As much as I've highlighted the importance of taking control of your own outcomes, too much control comes with its own disadvantages. If you overemphasize your internal locus of control, you may too quickly disregard an outsider's point of view. As Daniel Kahneman outlines in his book, *Thinking, Fast and Slow*, internalizing too much can make people susceptible to a phenomenon that he calls "What You See Is All There Is." It's a form of bias where you get overly caught up on only your side of the story and fail to see other points of views.

As you can imagine, this way of seeing the world can

create costly mistakes. You must consider alternative points of view if you want to make the best choices, especially if you are tasked with formulating business projections. Simply put, the best decision-makers are those who are supported by a diverse team of people who offer many different viewpoints. It is imperative that you have a good team in place, with members who feel comfortable sharing their opinions and views—even going so far as to try to poke holes in your proposed course of action. This will help you to avoid potential setbacks or obstacles when you implement your plans.

If you are too focused on your own control and your own views you may neglect what your competitors are doing. While it's generally a good idea to stay in your own lane and not pay much attention to what others are doing, you don't want to be caught completely off guard. Having a good team around you will prevent that from happening.

Above all else, it is imperative that you keep your ego in check. The bigger your ego, the less likely you will have a system of checks and balances like this in place. It's also less likely that you will take potential threats seriously. As with everything, there is a happy middle ground for all of these habits of success, and the most successful people know how to stay rooted in the middle.

Too much focus on your internal locus of control can also lead to some bizarre and irrational fears. Consider traveling by airplane versus traveling by car. Many people are afraid of flying because it's something they cannot control. They feel more comfortable and safer driving because they are controlling the car, even though statistical analysis proves that people are far more likely to be hurt or killed in an automobile accident than a plane crash.

A PRAGMATIC APPROACH

Because we are human, we are bound to focus on some elements outside of our control from time to time. Don't get discouraged if you find yourself doing this. Even the most successful people slip up every now and then. In fact, there are times when it's necessary to focus on external factors. "Overall, I remind myself not to worry about things outside of my control," says Navy SEAL Dan Luna. "I also think it is foolish to not consider something just because you cannot control it. Using mental energy to think about things outside of your control can assist you in your next step."

So the key is not to completely avoid spending energy on things you cannot control, but realizing when you're doing it. The sooner we realize that, the quicker we can get our minds back on track, focusing on the things we *can* control. Doing so will improve our mental state and also keep us on the road to success.

With a strong work ethic in place and a developed internal locus of control, you will be on the path to success. But the realization that you're the one who has to do the work—that ultimately, it's all on you—can be difficult to handle. As that reality sets in, it's easy to feel overwhelmed or pessimistic about how much you may be able to change. To be your most productive and to avoid doubts detracting from your success, you'll need a positive mindset.

PUTTING IT INTO PRACTICE

Keep a journal of your largest obstacles to overcome: By jotting down the challenges or setbacks that you faced each day and whether or not you had control over them, you'll begin to understand what outcomes you can control. Identifying that element of control will either focus your attention on solutions you can create, or it will reveal that those issues are out of your control. Knowing which issues are out of your control will allow you to focus your energy and attention on matters that *are* within your control.

—

CHAPTER 3

POSITIVE MINDSET

" —
Whether you think you can or think
you can't—you're right."

—HENRY FORD

TO UNDERSTAND THE IMPORTANCE of thinking positively, consider a patient who is battling cancer. If that patient stays upbeat and continues to think positively about their chances of defeating cancer, they'll convince themselves that they can do it. Subsequently, they'll set out to do everything in their power to control how they get better. They will strictly adhere to their medication protocol, they'll drink the right amount of fluids as directed by their medical care team, and they'll do their own research and reading to learn of other things that they can do to improve their chance of success. But if a patient adopts a negative mindset, they'll feel like a victim. They'll likely complain constantly, and they may begin to think that they won't get better. That can lead to that patient not adhering to the routines prescribed by their medical care team. Out of those two scenarios, which patient do you think has the better chance of beating cancer?

In his books *Learned Optimism* and *Flourish*, Martin Seligman asserts that optimistic people generally live healthier lives and are less prone to getting sick than people who adopt a pessimistic point of view. That's not to say that you can prevent cancer just by adopting a positive mindset, but it is a reminder that once you are presented with a challenging diagnosis, you have the choice as to how you perceive the situation and how you respond to it. You must not forget that *you* have the power to choose how you respond to any situation in which you find yourself.

Say you are in a car accident that is not your fault. You are not seriously injured. If you adopt a negative mindset, you'll feel like a victim. That will impact your mood, which will also impact how you treat your coworkers, friends, and family. Those negative interactions can put a strain on your personal life and they could also lead to troublesome situations at work. In this scenario, thinking negatively could be the catalyst of a downward spiral of emotions and interactions, all of which pull you further away from success. Alternatively, you can choose to be grateful that you were unharmed, which will make you feel more appreciation for being alive, for the job that you have, and for your family and friends. That is the power of mindset. It's choosing to have the right attitude, which is key in laying the foundation for your success. Without it, you'll end up on a path that only leads to mediocrity.

SELF-BELIEF

In the eighty-three years since it was written, Napolean Hill's *Think and Grow Rich* has steadily risen to become one of the most popular self-help books of all time. The overriding theme of the book is that you must first believe in yourself before you can achieve success. Without belief in yourself, the chances that you will take that first step in the right direction are slim. It might sound gimmicky but it's absolutely true—your ability to take action is powered by self-confidence.

Mindset isn't everything, of course. I might have the desire and the willpower to play in the NBA. I may even have a strong belief in my ability to do it, but skill and natural athleticism are two factors that also greatly contribute to my chances of becoming a professional basketball player. Nevertheless, the role that your mindset plays can be the difference maker when all other pivotal factors are accounted for. "Mind is everything," said Paavo Nurmi, a nine-time Olympic gold medalist and legendary Finnish distance runner. "All that I am, I am because of my mind."

Alex Hutchinson's book about human potential, *Endure: Mind, Body, and the Curiously Elastic Limits of Human Performance*, focuses on endurance athletes. It provides glimpses into the minds of successful runners and investigates how their self-belief leads them to success. Hutchinson explains that through high-intensity training, disciplined athletes can increase their pain tolerance. It stands to reason that if you are willing to spend hours and hours enduring pain, your mindset must be incredibly strong. In fact, Hutchinson further connects a positive mindset with success by revealing that many unproven Kenyan runners simply show up at dirt tracks in Kenya to train alongside some of the country's best runners. Not surprisingly, many of those Kenyans develop into elite runners themselves; that success stems from a level of self-belief that few others have.

We can point to many other sports examples as proof that self-belief and a positive mindset are difference makers. Until Roger Bannister broke the four-minute mark for the mile in track and field, many thought such a feat was impossible. Once Bannister accomplished it in 1954, however, other runners soon began running sub-four-minute miles themselves. In the book *Peak: Secrets from the New Science of Expertise*, authors Anders Ericcson and Robert Pool share a story about Gunder Hägg, a Swedish endurance athlete who trained on a homemade, 1,500-meter track and often had his father time his laps. As the story goes, his father one day sensed that his son was lacking motivation, so he told Hägg his time was four minutes and fifty seconds for the 1,500 meters. It was an impressive time, but it was also a lie. However, that false lap time provided Hägg with the added motivation and self-belief to keep training—and to train harder. He went on to set 15 world records in races ranging from 1,500 to 5,000 meters in length.

Conversely, the record that racing horse Secretariat set on a one-and-a-half-mile dirt track at the Belmont Stakes in 1973 is one that still stands and that many pundits expect will never be broken. It seems likely that horses do not have that same innate belief or knowledge that records exist and can be broken.

PLACEBO EFFECT

The placebo effect provides a good test for the power and influence of a person's mindset. It's also a topic of contentious debate within the scientific community. In many cases, taking placebos has produced positive effects even when patients weren't taking any real medicine. The exact mechanisms of how they work are still a mystery, but Professor Ted Kaptchuk of Harvard-affiliated Beth Israel Deaconess Medical Center believes they can work, albeit with limitations. "Placebos may make you feel better, but they will not cure you," he says. "They have been shown to be most effective for conditions like pain management, stress-related insomnia, and cancer treatment side effects like fatigue and nausea." In the same way that mindset will not make you the next Michael Jordan, the placebo effect only goes so far. But if taking nothing can make you feel better and reduce your discomfort, then that says a lot about the power of our mindset.

Author David Epstein in his book *Range: Why Generalists Triumph in a Specialized World* references a Finnish medical study during which doctors treated two groups of patients suffering from meniscus tears. Those in the first group underwent surgery to physically repair the tendon, while the other group received a "sham surgery"—they were taken to the operating room where incisions were made and then sewed back up, but no reparative work was done to the injured tendon. Interestingly, both groups of patients experienced similar recovery outcomes. Again, the placebo effect and self-belief will not guarantee success, but knowing and believing in yourself provides a foundation to get you started. It will help you build the momentum to make progress.

GROWTH MINDSET VS FIXED MINDSET

As a general rule, successful people share a similar mindset, one that is focused on self-improvement. These people constantly think about how they can improve every aspect of their lives. According to Carol Dweck in her book *Mindset: The New Psychology of Success*, these successful people possess a "growth mindset," which is the belief that abilities are not innate and that they can be enhanced. If you adopt a growth mindset and discover that you are not inherently good at something right away, you'll believe that you have the ability to improve. People with a growth mindset often seek out challenges that will allow them to learn and to grow, and they are generally more accepting of criticism and take inspiration from other people's success.

The opposite of a growth mindset is one that is fixed. People with fixed mindsets believe that their skills and intelligence are pre-determined and unalterable. They often avoid challenges because they assume they cannot succeed. Because of that, they are less likely to take risks. They also receive criticism poorly and feel threatened by others' success. Not surprisingly, a growth mindset is critical for success as it instills a perspective that embraces learning, adaptation, and evolution. If you don't have a growth mindset and belief in yourself, you won't be very likely to begin work on improving yourself.

Legendary business coach Art Turock believes that everything starts with mindset. According to Turock (as outlined in the book *Peak: Secrets from the New Science of Expertise*), if you believe that talents are innate, you will be easily convinced that you do not have the necessary skills or ability to succeed. If you believe that someone is smarter or more charismatic simply because they were born that way, you won't pursue the education or work on the skills that will improve those aspects of yourself. Turock advocates a growth mindset and believes that through deliberate practice in specific areas, people have the capability to improve.

From my own observation, people who adopt a growth mindset are less likely to let their egos get in the way of receiving constructive criticism. That creates a positive feedback loop, which provides a steady stream of advice and guidance, allowing them to adapt, improve, and to continually move closer to their goals.

FIXED ABILITIES

Much like the nature versus nurture debate, a question is often raised about mindset. Are you born with the abilities that you have, or can you train to be better and stronger? Although it's easy to get lost in this debate, nearly everyone agrees that it's a combination of the two. According to Drew Bailey, a psychologist at the University of California Irvine: "Without both genes and environments, there are no outcomes." In *The Sports Gene*, David Epstein references U.S. Olympic softball player Jennie Finch to make this point. Several years ago, Finch pitched to a variety of Major League Baseball players, striking each of them out. Even though those MLB players had incredible skill of their own, those skills did not immediately translate to a softball environment. (On softball fields the mound is positioned closer to home plate and the pitchers use a different wind-up, which means batters have to track the ball from a different release point than what they are familiar with if they play baseball.)

If it helps, think of people like personal computers. Athletes, as an example, are born with an inherent hardware component (genetics), but they still require the right software programming (experience, practice, and training) to be successful and to maximize the full potential of their hardware. I could have a work ethic stronger than that of any other living person, but without the right physical attributes and hardware, no amount of hard work will turn me into the next Kobe Bryant. In fact, if you look closely at Bryant and Michael Jordan—two of the greatest basketball players of all time—you'll notice that they were similarly sized and possess rare "hardware" (innate talent) along with a resolute work ethic. The combination of their hardware and software is what allowed them to become all-time greats.

Epstein also compares two champion high jumpers: Stefan Holm—who trained for much of his life—and Donald Thomas, who participated in track and field while in high school but then took years off before returning to the sport and experiencing almost immediate success. In Thomas's case, genetics overshadowed how much (or how little) he trained leading up to his success, but his past experience in high school still makes the case that preparation and training play at least some role in an individual's ability to succeed.

What does this all mean for mindset? It means that even if life gives you lemons, you can still make lemonade through a commitment to working hard and staying positive. You can choose to be optimistic about your abilities. And for those who do have the advantage of being born with plenty of natural ability, an optimistic mindset (combined with a dedication to practice) can lead to even greater success.

OPTIMISM

If you see an opportunity present itself, do you first think of what could go right? Or do you immediately think about everything that could go wrong? If you want to be successful, you're going to have to think a lot about what can go right, not the other way around. A successful mindset requires optimism in spades, especially if you have entrepreneurial ambitions.

Fortunately, the mind's explanatory style can be reconfigured through training, which means you can learn to be optimistic even if you don't currently think that way. Pessimists generally think of things in terms of the three Ps: permanent, pervasive, and personal. If you are a door-to-door salesman and a prospective client slams the door in your face, you'll believe it happened because of one of those three Ps—you might think that your skills are inferior and will never improve (permanent), you might think that you lack a strong personality whether in business or your social life (pervasive), or you might assume that it was something about you specifically that motivated that person to close the door (personal).

If you adopted an optimistic perspective, on the other hand, you'd reason that that person was just having a bad day. You wouldn't infer that the outcome of having the door slammed in your face was a reflection of you or what you did. It's easy to see which explanatory style and outlook will lead to more success, isn't it? The more optimistic you are, the better you'll be at shaking off failure and moving forward in the face of those challenges. A growth mindset and optimism go hand-in-hand. You cannot have one without the other.

Optimism can have a positive impact on more than just your success; it can also improve your health. In *Flourish*, author Martin Seligman recounts the results of studies that show that optimistic people are 25 percent less likely to have a second heart attack when compared to the baseline average, whereas pessimists are 25 percent more likely.

Optimism may not be all that we need, but it is a great place to start. According to Gabriele Oettingen, who has studied optimism extensively, thinking optimistically is only beneficial if those thoughts are still rooted in reality. She coined the term WOOP (Wish, Outcome, Obstacle, Plan) as a good way to build upon dreams. The third O—obstacle—is key, since it requires people to consider the hurdles in their paths and to create a plan to overcome them. That dose of realism will help you to better manage your expectations; it will guide your work ethic and allow you to set more realistic goals.

SELF-DOUBT

Even if you are an optimist and choose to view the glass as half full, you may still be burdened with self-doubt. Nearly everyone experiences self-doubt, but balancing it with at least equal portions of self-confidence is crucial. In fact, having some self-doubt can be a good thing. It can improve our relationships, since a person with some self-doubt is going to put more emphasis on getting along with others. It can also keep our egos from growing too large or our confidence in our abilities from getting out of hand. After all, if you are overconfident, you'll be less likely to prepare as long or as hard as is needed. If you think that you can just show up and crush the competition, you're likely not going to spend the extra time in the gym or at the office. Having a bit of self-doubt can help counter this so that you strike the right balance between being under– and over-prepared.

Of course, too much self-doubt is deadly to success because it can prevent action. And without action, ideas remain just that—ideas. Even great ideas mean nothing without action, so it's important to be aware of your self-doubt and to understand the role that it is playing. If it's preventing you from taking action, you must eliminate it.

OPTIMISM BIAS

Optimism may be what you are striving for, but as is the case with many things in life, a dichotomy exists between too much and too little. What you are striving for is the perfect amount of positivity. You must balance optimism with a hint of caution. If you're too optimistic, you can develop a belief that you are less likely to be impacted by a negative or challenging event. This unrealistic way of thinking is known as optimism bias and it can manifest itself in various forms.

In *Thinking, Fast and Slow* Daniel Kahneman introduces an optimism bias known as the planning fallacy. Ultimately, it's an underestimation of the amount of time and resources that will be required to complete a given project. It can often impact entrepreneurs, and it's something that I (and my team) at Renaissance Periodization experienced during the development of the RP Diet App. Something we thought would take months or maybe a year actually took multiple years, and we encountered numerous setbacks and suffered plenty of failures along the way.

There's another equally harmful optimism bias known as the sunk-cost fallacy. Simply explained, this is a person's tendency to stay loyal to a behavior or endeavor based on the amount of time, energy, and/or money that they initially invested in it. I made this mistake with RP by sticking with a particular software program, despite the fact that it was inefficient for some aspects of our business. In particular, customer orders didn't always go through the system, but after a while I just learned to deal with it because the thought of switching to a completely new software and transferring all of the customer data that we had accrued was overwhelming. Eventually, we had to build a custom website that allowed us to sell and deliver products directly to consumers. As I learned, there comes a time when the right course of action is to admit defeat, regardless of the amount of time or money that has been spent.

If you have investors or a board of directors, a healthy dose of optimism is just what they want. Nobody who invests their money and/or time into a project will be happy or will continue to invest if that project's leader is pessimistic or lacks confidence. In those circumstances, being optimistic is incredibly beneficial. Just be sure you don't fall victim to an optimism bias.

GOAL SETTING

Yes, it's important to set goals. But just like optimism, there are pitfalls to goal setting. The first one is what psychologists describe as false-hope syndrome, and it pertains to setting goals—sometimes lofty goals—without factoring in the amount of hard work and dedication that will be required to achieve them. This syndrome lures people into a false sense of confidence. For example, you may want to lose 50 pounds, which is a fantastic goal that many people would benefit from. But that goal can very easily become unrealistic if you don't set a feasible time frame in which you can accomplish it. If you set a goal of losing 50 pounds in a couple of months, you'll likely be overwhelmed by the amount of hard work and dedication that will be required to lose that much weight in that short a period of time (if it can be done safely at all). In that state of being over-whelmed, you are much more likely to give up. The down-side here is not that the goals are too ambitious, but that the failure to reach them quickly discourages people early on and leaves them feeling like the pursuit is hopeless.

Behavioral economists have expanded on this idea by creating the hot-cold empathy gap. The "hot" refers to a person's emotional state and the desire to immediately satisfy urges. The "cold" state reflects someone's analytical side, which logically deduces the best course of action but does so without giving credence to the power of desire. In the book *Nudge: Improving Decisions about Health, Wealth and Happiness*, authors Richard Thaler and Cass Sun-stein set up a dinner party scene to illustrate this point. If a bowl of cashews is left out on the counter before din-ner, party guests may snack on them to the point that they ruin their appetite. That's being in a hot state. If they were to think about the dinner party days before, those same guests might decide not to snack on anything ahead of the meal. That's an easy decision to make at that time, but it becomes much harder to follow through on once hunger is introduced and snacks are readily available. It is easy to set goals and to make proclamations for yourself when you are thinking logically and rationally. But it becomes much harder when you must battle your emotions, especially once primal urges want to take over.

Still, you shouldn't shy away from setting really big goals. Lofty goals can play a positive role in creating your sense of identity and determining your purpose. Jim Col-lins, in his book *Built to Last: Successful Habits of Vision-ary Companies*, calls them "Big Hairy Audacious Goals" (or BHAGs). These far-reaching goals will help you to set the standard for yourself and/or your company and they'll serve as a catalyst for you taking action. If your goal is to run a company that holds a majority of the market share in a new field, for example, that overall goal will guide your company's vision and the actions that it will take. That over-arching goal will make it easier for you to create sub-goals, which will guide you down the path to eventual success. Think of it like a road trip. Your BHAGs are your final destination, but smaller goals (set weekly or monthly) are the turn-by-turn navigation that your GPS system provides. Accomplishing those sub-goals builds positive momentum and fuels your motivation to accomplish the larger goals that you've set. Just remember that too many sub-goals can be detrimental; if not held in check, those daily tasks might prevent you from accomplishing the bigger-picture objectives that you have to meet.

George T. Doran created an acronym to help people in setting objectives. He called it SMART (Specific, Measurable, Attainable, Relevant, and Time-bound). If you want to be successful, it is paramount that you set goals that fit the SMART acronym. Be sure that those goals make sense to you whether you are in a hot or cold state. If your goals pass the SMART filter, you are on the right track. Think of it as a checklist:

- Are your goals specific to what you are trying to achieve? If you want to run a mile in less than five minutes, for example, it makes sense to set goals that cover how many miles you should run per week and what you should eat to maximize your performance.
- Can you accurately measure your goals? This is import-

ant, since it allows you to understand if you are progressing. If you want to bench press 315 pounds, for example, you should measure how many sets and how many reps you perform during each workout, and the weight that you're lifting each time.

- Can you actually attain your goals? If they are realistically achievable, your goals will be much more appealing.
- Do your goals really matter to you? Are they relevant? It is important to set goals that align with *your* values and *your* purpose. Do not set goals for yourself that will only please or benefit someone else.
- How long will it take you to achieve your goals? Do not fall victim to false-hope syndrome and oversell yourself. If you have a large, imposing goal, you will be better off breaking that goal up into smaller sub-goals. You may want to lose 100 pounds, for example, but you'll be discouraged if you think that you can achieve that in a few months. Instead, set a goal to lose 10 pounds every six to eight weeks.

EGO

If we know that a growth mindset leads to more success, why would anyone be resistant to outside opinions or unreceptive to constructive criticism? It's because our egos get in the way. As author Ryan Holiday succinctly states, "Ego is the enemy." A big ego prevents people from listening to feedback, accepting criticism with an open mind, or working as hard as their goals require them to. It also leads to a self-serving bias.

Imagine that you're driving your car and you get passed

or cut off by someone driving recklessly and much too fast. If you're anything like me, you'll immediately proclaim that person to be a terrible driver. That's a common, real-world example of the self-serving bias. It's a way of thinking that attributes another person's faults or mistakes to their ability level, but their successes to luck. Similarly, that bias would lead someone to attribute his or her own success to their skill and their failures to bad luck. In the driving example, that "reckless" driver might be rushing home to a sick child or to the hospital for a family emergency. When working under a self-serving bias, you might not consider that possibility.

When you suffer from a self-serving bias you inevitably devote less time to developing and cultivating your skills. During RP's early years, I was working *in* the business much too often (instead of working on the business), and my ego prevented me from devoting time and energy to improving as a business owner. Had I reduced the size of my ego, I would have learned earlier and could have set up the business for greater success. Be careful in over-attributing success to your skill level. You must stay committed to the process of self-improvement.

To reduce the size of your ego, you must detach yourself from the situation. In other words, don't let emotions get the best of you. Train yourself to step back and look at the situation objectively. Once you set your emotions aside you will be more able to see things for what they are. In turn, you'll make the correct choices in regards to what needs to be corrected or improved.

By limiting the size of your ego, you'll also be more equipped to accept the blame for mistakes that you or your team members have made. Taking ownership of those problems is a critical piece of the puzzle. It will allow you to find solutions to those problems and to further prevent them from happening in the future. A small ego will also allow you to deflect praise onto your partners and/or colleagues. Not only will this improve morale, it will also reinforce the notion that you are smart—you've proven it by hiring even smarter people to work for you.

BRAIN FOOD

To develop a healthy and positive mindset, you must be judicious about what you're consuming. This pertains to what you feed your body *and* what you feed your mind. As you likely know, nutrition plays a key role in maximizing a person's physical performance and abilities. Without going into too much detail, your body will function at its best if your diet is comprised mostly of lean protein sources (meats, low-fat dairy, fish/seafood, eggs, and soy-based alternatives); healthy fats (nuts, nut butters, avocado, olive oil, and coconut oil—in moderation, of course); and healthy carbohydrates (fruits and vegetables, whole grains, and rice). Once you know what you should be feeding your body—for more information, refer to *The Renaissance Diet 2.0*—you should also understand what you should be feeding your mind.

The term "brain food" doesn't mean that certain foods will improve your mindset. Instead, it refers to the things that we expose our minds to. The most successful people feed their minds with content that enriches their lives or allows them to grow as human beings. In other words, they focus on things that are educational or beneficial. Social media, movies, and television programs aimed solely at entertainment don't make the list. That doesn't mean that you should avoid them altogether—those outlets are fine in moderation—but be careful what you're consistently feeding your mind. If you are constantly engaging in negativity, that brain food could shape your explanatory style and promote a more pessimistic outlook. Elevate your mind and you will elevate yourself in the process!

By now you understand why you must be a hard worker and that you—and only you—can put in that work. You also know what you can control and what is beyond your control. And when it comes to the things you can control, you recognize that you must be carefully optimistic and ready to work with a growth mindset.

Even though you have that understanding and are prepared to think positively, the journey that you must take to be successful will likely be strewn with obstacles and challenges. To be frank, the journey will be difficult. To get through it, you'll need to be disciplined.

PUTTING IT INTO PRACTICE

Keep a journal of at least three good things that happen to you each day: Making note of the positive aspects of your life on a daily basis will not only help you to develop gratitude and appreciation for them, it will also help to keep things in perspective. It's human nature to dwell on the negative things that we experience; too often we easily overlook the positive. By purposely identifying those favorable things—and writing them down—you'll begin to train yourself to see and appreciate the positives when they occur.

CHAPTER 4

DISCIPLINE

" —
Discipline is the bridge between
goals and accomplishment."

—JIM ROHN

IT'S EASY TO TALK ABOUT having the right mindset or focusing only on the things that you can control, but it's another matter to put them into action. I learned this for myself earlier this year as Lori battled breast cancer and endured chemotherapy treatments, all while we were subjected to months of quarantine due to the global pandemic caused by COVID-19. It was a challenging time, to say the least. As I learned, keeping a positive mindset and focusing only on the things that you can control requires more than just an understanding of those concepts. This is where discipline comes into play.

I was raised by two incredibly hard-working parents, and through that upbringing—and also possibly genetics—I grew up with a strong work ethic, understanding that hard work pays off. But I learned about discipline (and its importance) firsthand as a cross-country runner during the summer between my freshman and sophomore years of high school. I wasn't a particularly strong runner as a freshman, and I didn't make the varsity team. At the end of the school year, our coach gave the team its summer marching orders. We were to run 100 miles over the course of the summer, which would strengthen us for the start of the fall season. I focused on completing that objective, and when I returned to school in the fall I found myself able to keep pace with the top runners on the team from the year before. There was no secret to my improvement—it was my discipline and the hard work that I put in to log those miles. As it turns out, no one else on the team had run a full 100 miles over the summer.

That was a lightbulb moment for me. I realized that if I worked hard and did what others would not, I could perform as well or even better than them. More recently, in reading the book *Extreme Ownership: How U.S. Navy SEALs Lead and Win* by retired Navy SEALs Jocko Willink and Leif Babin, I experienced another epiphany. According to the authors, "discipline equals freedom." In fact, they acknowledge that the most successful people that they've worked with also happen to be the most disciplined. That connection is no coincidence.

But discipline is still difficult to maintain. There is a reason that many people only talk of being successful. It's easy to talk about the things you want to achieve when you're not putting in the work to achieve them. It's another thing entirely to put in the work to reach those goals.

MOTIVATION

Many people wrongly assume that inspiration and motivation are what drive people in the pursuit of their goals. While they are both great attributes that are necessary to take initial action, both are short-lived. It's often easy to find inspiration, and while that inspiration can be the spark that lights a fire to get you going, those feelings of inspiration can quickly fade. A healthy dose of motivation can usually pick up the slack, but nobody is motivated all the time. The thing that differentiates successful people from the masses is discipline. It's the commitment to do what is necessary no matter what.

Just to reiterate, unwavering motivation isn't necessary for success. You'd like to be motivated all of the time, of course, and that's something that people strive for, but it's often wrongly assumed that you must be motivated all the time if you're going to be successful. World-class athletes, just like beginners, struggle with motivation sometimes. It's good practice to seek out sources of inspiration and motivation—they'll always be helpful—but the key is to use the initial spark that those sources provide to develop a system of habits that can help you to stay disciplined. Don't be discouraged on days when you're lacking motivation— instead, rely on your self-discipline to carry you through.

Think of all the times when you knew that you should do something—a workout or a business-related task, for example—but you just couldn't find the drive to do it. Now imagine that in those same instances, you could summon an inner power that allowed you to complete that task. That's not motivation; that's discipline. Discipline is the attribute that keeps you motivated, and learning how to hone in on self-discipline is as close to a superpower as anyone will ever have. Remember, being successful requires traveling down a difficult road, one where hard work is required at every turn. Self-discipline is what's needed to get you to the finish line at the end of that road.

LONG-TERM THINKING
Imagine that someone places a warm, delicious doughnut

in front of you. If you're like many people, you'd probably waste little time taking a bite and then thoroughly enjoying the rest of it, too. But now imagine that you are overweight and your doctor has advised you to lose at least 20 pounds. Do you succumb to the temptation and devour the doughnut, in the process moving further away from your goal? Or, do you think of the long-term consequences that come with the choices that you make in the here and now? We are all human and susceptible to urges that offer immediate gratification; however, those who can withstand those urges and focus on the bigger picture are more likely to find success. In fact, a longitudinal study in New Zealand revealed that people who possessed more self-control (and thereby, more discipline) were healthier and more financially secure. They even had better teeth.

On the topic of teeth, I used to dread going to the dentist. My wife, on the other hand, was never worried about it. Of course, my wife also took great care of her teeth, using an electric toothbrush twice a day and regularly flossing. I did neither of those things. After one particularly rough dentist appointment, I decided to mimic my wife. I began using an electric toothbrush and I flossed daily. Not surprisingly, this newfound discipline improved the health of my teeth, which made future trips to the dentist much less stressful.

As you may have already guessed, all of this means that the ability to think long-term is paramount to success. Let's say you're running a business. You know that your reputation means everything. Furthermore, you know that sending the right message to consumers is a critical piece of the formula. If you receive an offer from a company that is willing to pay you thousands of dollars each month to promote its product, would you take it? If you automatically answer yes, you might be in trouble. Let's say the company's product isn't trustworthy, or there is little evidence that the product delivers on its promise. Your endorsement of it could negatively reflect on your own reputation. If you are swayed by the immediate gratification of thousands of dollars each month, you could be setting yourself up for long-term failure.

Take youth sports in this country as another example. Many American parents think that their children need to specialize in a sport from a young age, that this will be the key to their children developing into professional athletes someday. It also provides some immediate gratification for both the parents and the children; those kids, given their focus on only one sport, will likely be the best players on their respective teams. In reality, a focus on early specialization has been shown to increase the chances of injury. It has also been proven to produce less successful long-term results since the kids are more likely to burn out at some point along the way. Marv Marinovich, for example, prepared his son, Todd, to play football, going so far as to control almost every aspect of Todd's life—the young football player was never allowed to eat fast food, even as a child! Todd earned a scholarship to play quarterback at the University of Southern California and was later selected by the Oakland Raiders in the first round of the 1991 NFL draft. He certainly enjoyed short-term success in his younger years. Soon after Todd entered the NFL, however, he developed a substance abuse problem, and within three years he was out of the league entirely.

It would be easy to misinterpret the Marinovich family's story as a cautionary tale about being too disciplined. After all, Marv made choices early in his sons' life that were influenced by a long-term goal. Yet, Marv was too focused on his son being a great football player. He was seduced by the immediate gratification of watching his son play better than any of the kids around him. Remember, a parent's ultimate goal is to ensure their children's long-term success and happiness. Marv let his son's immediate success derail him from making decisions that would ensure Todd's best possible future.

Some of today's most accomplished athletes are successful because they don't lose focus on their long-term goals. "I realize that not every day will be a great day, but every day is an opportunity to get closer to where I want to be, whether I'm motivated or not," says Annie Thorisdottir. "If you only work hard on the days where you feel like it, you will not experience progress long term."

GRIT

If you're going to stay dedicated to your long-term goals, you'll need to be disciplined. In other words, you're going to need grit—strength of character, perseverance, and passion for your long-term goals. There's no better term or definition to support this chapter on self-discipline.

Grit and a positive explanatory outlook go hand in hand. That relationship is something that Angela Duckworth extrapolates on in her aptly titled book *Grit: The Power of Passion and Perseverance*. It is difficult to persevere and to think about the long term if you aren't optimistic that you can reach your goals. Having grit is having the ability to look failure in the face, get back up, and keep going after setbacks or failures. It is the relentless pursuit of your goals, holding those long-term goals in such high regard that you are willing to do just about anything to reach them.

If and when you fail, you must have a growth mindset and a positive explanatory style. You must consider any obstacle that you encounter as a learning point, as a way to improve. There is a lot to be said about simply outworking your competition. Being gritty sums that up. If you are committed to daily improvements and you cultivate a mindset that supports that endeavor, you've got plenty of grit.

Gritty individuals show up to practice early with an open mind. They are committed to their long-term goals and are willing to put in however much time and practice is required to learn and improve. "I may not always have the strongest or best mindset, but I always push through or bounce back regardless," says Mattie Rogers, a national champion and world-medalist weightlifter. "A lot of it is an unwillingness to settle for anything less than all of my effort, and that carries me through even the roughest days.

"There are almost more days I don't necessarily feel like training or eating as I should than days where I do," she continues, "so it's just learning to be uncomfortable and do things I may not want to do."

In *Flourish*, Martin Seligman references studies on grit that were conducted by Duckworth. She concluded that a person's grittiness—their ability and willingness to buckle down and to stay committed to a task—was more important than their level of intelligence. People with lower IQs but more grit regularly outperformed those who had higher IQs but less grit. Those studies reinforce a popular saying that we now know to be true: hard work beats talent when talent doesn't work hard.

DELIBERATE PRACTICE

Imagine that you want to take up a new sport, like golf. How would you choose to pursue that new interest? You could visit the driving range on your own to hit balls and hopefully (but not assuredly) get better. You could schedule a few social rounds of golf with some friends. Or you could find a swing coach and schedule lessons to target specific areas of your game. Many people would opt for the first two choices, but if you really want to excel as a golfer (especially if you're new to the sport), the third option provides the only avenue to do it.

The act of getting better—no matter what activity or endeavor—requires not just practice, but deliberate practice. As outlined in the book *Peak: Secrets from the New Science of Expertise* by Anders Ericsson and Robert Pool, deliberate practice differs from ordinary practice in seven important ways:

1. It usually requires an objective way to measure performance and track the standouts.
2. It requires a coach who can take you further using training that is defined by purpose and meaning. Using our golf analogy, if you are only hitting balls at the range on your own, you likely won't get much better, even if you practice a lot. You need specific guidance from a coach to give you direction on ways to improve.
3. Deliberate practice pushes you outside of your comfort zone.

4. It relies on clearly defined goals and objectives for each practice session.

5. It includes timely feedback on where you can improve.

6. It trains you to create mental representations. Over time, this will allow you to monitor yourself internally, which means you won't need as much external coaching as you might have in the beginning.

7. Deliberate practice allows you to develop new and specific skills that enhance the ability you already have.

If that sounds like a lot, it's because it *is* a lot! In fact, this type of deliberate practice requires so much energy and focus that even the most successful athletes and performers in the world typically only practice this way for a handful of hours each day, at the most. Deliberate practice is hard—that's why so many people resign themselves to just being "good enough," instead of working to be the very best that they can be.

DISCIPLINE CARRYOVER

Self-discipline is most commonly associated with health and fitness, but it can be applied to—and positively impact—many other facets of your life. You can learn to be more disciplined financially, for example, limiting the types of purchases that provide instant gratification but ultimately get in the way of you saving more or improving yourself. Instead of buying designer clothes, for example, you could invest that money in a retirement fund, or you could enroll in a weekend course to learn a new skill or strengthen one that you already have.

If you apply discipline to your spending habits, you'll

be better equipped for retirement—and better equipped to resist the allure of persuasive advertising campaigns aimed at convincing you to spend money . . . most often on frivolous things. In *The Willpower Instinct: How Self-Control Works, Why It Matters, and What You Can Do to Get More of It*, author Kelly McGonigal, a leading researcher at Stanford University, urges readers to imagine their future selves. As she acknowledges, human beings are notoriously bad at delaying immediate gratification. But if we can envision ourselves in the future, she says, we can make better decisions for the long term. In fact, financial institutions are now employing this same technique, which encourages their clients to invest more into their retirements. In *The Millionaire Next Door: The Surprising Secrets of America's Wealthy*, Thomas J. Stanley and William D. Danko provide even more motivation to be disciplined with your finances. According to Stanley, many of the millionaires in the United States didn't inherit their wealth or strike it rich with a brilliant new product, company, or service. Instead, through disciplined spending habits, they were able to save and invest, slowly accumulating their wealth.

Discipline doesn't just enhance our fitness, nutrition, or financial regiments; it can also significantly impact our emotions. In fact, in their book *Emotional Intelligence 2.0*, authors Travis Bradberry and Jean Greaves suggest that having control of your emotions is as vital to success as overall intelligence. Many successful people have higher-than-average IQs, but Bradberry and Greaves acknowledge that success also stems from effective interactions with other people.

Consider a business scenario where you must work with

an unlikable boss or colleague. That person's negative personality traits—whatever they might be—are certain to make the prospect of working with them more challenging. But if you are self-aware and if you can control your emotions, you'll limit the number of negative interactions that occur between you and that unlikable colleague or boss. Keeping your emotions in check will prevent arguments from forming and that, by itself, will prevent you from possibly squandering away opportunities for greater advancement.

Being emotionally disciplined will also help you to make better long-term choices. In particular, it will help you to avoid making rash decisions. Let's say you're running a business and a major competitor in your industry launches a new product. If you overreact to that news and make hasty decisions to respond in some way, that could weaken your company and its position in the marketplace, not strengthen it. Emotional overreaction, especially from someone in a leadership role, can be construed as a sign of weakness. If you panic, chances are the people who work for you will, too. And if no one is thinking logically or rationally, your company could be headed for significant trouble.

The more you can slow yourself down and use your rational mind, the better off you will be. By stepping back from a situation before engaging in any emotional responses, you'll have time to evaluate the scenario. This allows the executive functioning part of your brain—the human aspect of the brain—to take over for the more animalistic part of the brain, which is reactionary. Letting the executive functioning part of your brain do the heavy lifting whenever you need to make decisions that impact both the long-term and the short-term outcomes is always a wise strategy. Implementing this type of approach will also train you to become more aware of your emotions. Self-awareness leads to better self-management, and if you can better manage your emotions, you'll make better decisions overall.

HABITS OR SHORTCUTS?

For worthwhile endeavors, shortcuts simply do not exist. It's clear now that discipline is hard; however, there are ways to make it a little easier. That assistance takes the form of establishing habits. "Successful people aren't born that way," says author Don Marquis. "They become successful by establishing the habit of doing things unsuccessful people do not like to do. The successful people do not always like doing these things themselves, they just get on and do them."

The first time we work to complete any new task, our brains are working harder than normal to process all of the information that is required to do that work. Over time, as we repeat the steps necessary to complete that task, the brain begins to automate the process. This forms the basis of a habit, and those habits allow us to be more efficient with our energy usage throughout the day.

Habits are essentially made up of three parts, the most important of which is the cue. A cue triggers the brain to turn on autopilot. To use a dieting analogy, if you always look in your pantry as you walk by it, that glance can signal the start of a familiar routine, which might be to grab a handful of the unhealthy snack that you most enjoy—a hyperpalatable food (food that tastes really good), which provides immediate gratification. To change a habit, you need to replace the routine with something else. In this particular example, you'll want to replace the hyperpalatable food choice with something healthier. There needs to be something there to help fill that void, but choosing a better alternative creates a win/win situation.

To take a more extreme approach, you can eliminate the temptation altogether. In this pantry example, that would mean not buying the unhealthy foods that you typically snack on. Not having those foods accessible will weaken the initial cue (it might eliminate it completely). At that point, the whole sequence can be bypassed. On the flip side, if you want to create a new habit of flossing your teeth regularly, you can improve your chances of succeeding by putting the floss somewhere you will easily see it every day. The more you can simplify and make your habits easier, the less willpower you will have to exert. And since our willpower is limited each day, creating these habits conserves our mental capacity, which allows us to do more and to direct that willpower toward more important tasks.

Staying disciplined and sticking to the process of creating new habits is hard work, but you can make it easier on yourself through pre-commitment. If you want to start working out early in the morning, for example, you'll obviously want to set an alarm (probably a second one, too), but you can also lay out your gym clothes next to your bed the night before, which will make it easier for you to get going in the morning. As another example, planning and prepping meals for the week is a great way to help you stick to a diet. If you have a prepped meal for you at work, it will be easier to eat what you're supposed to rather than navigating the challenges that come with going out for lunch—challenges that include social pressures from friends or coworkers and the alluring sights and smells of delicious (but unhealthy) food. And if you struggle with time management at work, you can create a daily schedule where you reserve a block of time to answer emails, or you can devote an hour for you to focus on the most important tasks that day. We are all human, and when left to our own devices we can struggle with staying on track. Preparing like this ahead of time will make things easier.

Aristotle believed that we are what we repeatedly do. "Excellence, then," echoed Will Durant, an American historian and philosopher, "is not an act, but a habit."

Being disciplined—and staying disciplined— is ridiculously hard, but developing habits over time will allow you to reduce the amount of mental energy that is needed to stay on task and to do the right things. Remarkably, the human brain represents only 2 percent of the body's total size, but it uses almost 20 percent of the body's total energy. Creating beneficial habits will allow you to put the majority of that energy consumption to good use.

TOO MUCH DISCIPLINE

Just like the behavioral skills that we have discussed in previous chapters, there can be a downside to having too much discipline. This is most often seen and most easily understood in the world of fitness. It takes discipline to stick to a workout routine, especially a vigorous one, but if you are too rigid in terms of your discipline, you could push past your own limits and wind up injuring yourself. If you are so disciplined, for example, that you *must* work out every day, it is likely that you won't allow yourself enough recovery time.

My colleagues Dr. Mike Israetel and Dr. James Hoffmann coined the term "Maximum Recoverable Volume" (MRV). They deduced that there is a healthy limit to how much fitness training one body can endure. Your MRV is the maximum amount of work you can do while still properly recovering. Calculating MRV requires documenting training sessions that slowly increase in intensity. Once performance dips, training intensity is greatly reduced until the athlete feels fully recovered, at which point the process repeats itself, only at a slightly higher intensity at the start. After three or four cycles, patterns will emerge that determine the best estimate of an athlete's current MRV.

Personally, I am someone who often pushes myself to the limits, sometimes past what I thought my limits were. If you operate in a similar way, you must be smart and acknowledge when you've reached existing limits. Only then can you make the choice to consciously push past them with an understanding of the possible risks involved. You can also be overly disciplined in business. If you impose strict checklists or guides that all employees must follow, you may be limiting your team's potential. Having goals or quotas that must be met can sometimes backfire, since they introduce incentives that aren't always in the best interest of the company. For example, if you offer a bonus to each member of the sales team that reaches a threshold value, some of those salespeople might stoop to unethical tactics, including competing against their colleagues, instead of working with their colleagues for the betterment of everyone and the company as a whole.

As chronicled in *The Impulse Society: America in the Age of Instant Gratification* by Paul Roberts, it's not uncommon to see this playing out at venture capital firms, where the more immediate interests of board members and investors looking for a return on their financial backing can clash with the business strategies of slow and gradual growth. Incidentally, those strategies for measured growth over a longer period of time carry the best odds for long-term success. It's another example of the risks that come with seeking immediate gratification.

Much like how over-training can lead to injury, too much discipline in business can also lead to burnout. Being successful absolutely requires a tenacious work ethic—and many times an almost obsessive passion for your desired goals—but being able to focus on yourself at times to recharge the batteries is equally necessary.

You can even have too much grit, which David Epstein reveals in his book *Range: Why Generalists Triumph in a Specialized World*. According to Epstein, Army cadets who commit much of their time and energy to the military can often feel overly committed to staying in the Army, even if they learn that they are better suited for a different career path. The same can be said for sinking too many resources into a specific goal, which ties back into the sunk-cost fallacy. Not surprisingly, people who have too much grit are more apt to suffer from this form of bias.

Just remember, you must walk a fine line between having too much of something and not enough. Finding that right balance is crucial, even when it comes to your own self-discipline. Telltale signs that your discipline is getting in the way of success include feeling overtired all of the time, general irritability, and frequent injuries. If any of these things begin to define how you feel or act for days on end, you would be better served dialing things back and allowing yourself to rest and recover.

A PRAGMATIC VIEW

There will be times when you are motivated to face your struggles and obstacles head on, and there will be days when you'd much rather take the path of least resistance. All successful people experience these conflicting emotions, including the world's best athletes. Many people believe that champion athletes don't experience days of low motivation. I can tell you from my own experiences as a coach that they most certainly do. What distinguishes them from the masses is their ability to keep going and to push through, even on days when they don't feel like it.

The most successful people in all facets of life have learned that they simply need to convince themselves to take the first step toward positive action. It can be a literal step in the direction of the gym or it can be reaching for a healthy snack in the fridge versus an unhealthy one. Just getting started is usually enough to carry you through the difficult tasks that lay ahead. "I find that the days that I don't feel like training often end up being the days I get the best workouts in," reveals Nita Strauss, an RP athlete and one of the world's best rock guitarists. "I make a deal with myself that I will get dressed, go to the gym and do 10 minutes of cardio. If, after that, I'm still not feeling it, then I'll go home. Once I am there and doing it, it sticks. I haven't gone home early from a workout yet."

At this point it might seem that you have all the tools in place to be successful. You're committed to working hard. You understand that you should only focus on the things you can control. You've trained yourself to think optimistically, to establish a growth mindset, and to not let your ego get in the way. And you've learned that you're going to need a lot of discipline, but you've also learned that there are ways to strengthen that dedication.

There is something that you're still missing. It's a commitment to learning and adhering to your purpose. After all, you can work hard and do everything right, but if you don't know why you're doing it you won't get very far. Remember, success doesn't come from working hard on just *anything*, it comes from working hard on very specific things and for a very specific reason. Only that reason will allow you to know which specific things are worthy of your attention and the subsequent hard work that you will devote to them.

PUTTING IT INTO PRACTICE

Make specific plans for the goals that you want to accomplish and the habits that you want to create. It's important that you make detailed plans for the actions that you want to take. Committing to those details will hold you accountable, and they'll make it easier for you to develop better discipline. For example, if you want to start a new fitness program, it's not enough to say, "I'll go to the gym tomorrow." You must be more detailed than that. Pick a specific time. Say: "I'll work out at 3:00 p.m. tomorrow. I will pack my gym bag ahead of time and will take it with me to the office." Those details will make it easier for you to following through on that commitment.

CHAPTER 5

PURPOSE
& MEANING

IN TODAY'S WORLD, we live better than at any other point in human history. We have more wealth, more prosperity, and the ability to live longer and healthier lives than ever before. Yet, Viktor Frankl, in the quote on the previous page, hits the nail on the head. Despite all of our advancements, people seem to be in poorer health as far as their mental well-being is concerned. Sure, we can enjoy quick fixes of happiness from good food, new possessions, or advancements in technology, but those bursts of positive emotion are fleeting. Remember that Martin Seligman's PERMA recipe for happiness (positive emotion, engagement, relationships, meaning, and achievement/accomplishment) depends on both "meaning" and "achievement." True happiness is rooted in a person's sense of purpose and the achievements that they make by doing what they love to do.

Before you convince yourself that making lots of money will provide you with a lifetime of happiness, consider Daniel Gilbert's discovery (outlined in his book *Stumbling on Happiness*) that once a person is financially stable enough to cover their basic needs, the additional money that they make or acquire doesn't bring them additional happiness.

Based on Gilbert's research and the studies that he conducted, the old saying that money can't buy happiness is true. This is not to say that making more money doesn't conjure positive emotions, but making more money typically requires more time spent working. And at some point, too much work can be a negative, as it eats away at the time that you could be devoting to other aspects of your life that provide a healthy balance, like spending time with friends and family, for example.

PURPOSE

Simon Sinek champions the idea that every person has the right to fulfillment, that experiencing that sense of fulfillment is something that everyone can control. It's not by chance, he argues, that people achieve that emotional state. "Every single one of us," he writes in *Find Your Why*, "is entitled to feel fulfilled by the work we do, to wake up feeling inspired to go to work . . . and to return home with a sense that we contributed to something larger than ourselves." When you start with a larger overall purpose, Sinek reveals, that purpose draws others in. By and large, this is a good thing; after all, we have all found inspiration before. Successful individuals have the ability to inspire others, to convince people to follow them in their mission and to be a part of something bigger than themselves. When you create this atmosphere it draws out the best in others. People who are inspired and motivated to be a part of something special are more likely to enjoy the work that is required, and that enjoyment also means that they'll put in their greatest effort and produce their best work.

Rock guitarist Nita Strauss reveals a similar calling.

"I'm fueled by the desire to make a new path where there wasn't one before, succeed while inspiring others, and getting to do what I love," she says.

A crucial component in striking a good balance between time spent on things that you enjoy and time spent working is to find a profession that doesn't feel like work. You've likely heard that a key to being happy is finding a career that appeals to you, to truly love what you do. That is generally true. In fact, it's best to think about things in this way: a job is merely something that people have and do to make a living; a career can best be defined as a person's focused line of work, something that drives them to be successful; but a "calling" is something that provides people an outlet to find their true meaning and purpose in life. A calling becomes part of your identity.

Even if you love your job, there will be days—possibly many of them—when it will feel like work. On those days you might not glean much enjoyment from the tasks that you perform, but you'll be more inclined to put in the work to get them done if you harbor a passion for what you do and you understand your overall mission. You'll still need to be disciplined, but that passion and your purpose are crucial to success.

Entrepreneurs are impacted in this way more so than many other businesspeople. In the beginning, their passion for the enterprise that they wish to create is what drives them, but as they progress and as that initial idea takes shape, the amount of work that is required to see it through becomes monumental. It's not uncommon for many entrepreneurs to teeter on the brink of burnout, but through a focus on their bigger purpose, by and large they see the project through. All of this to say, you can work 80-hour weeks, but if you don't believe in what you're doing, those 80-hour work weeks will soon feel like too much of a burden and not worth the commitment.

Elon Musk effectively describes what it's like to be an entrepreneur. "Running a start-up is like eating glass and staring into the abyss," he says. Needless to say, that doesn't sound like much fun, which is why any successful entrepreneur needs a strong sense of purpose to keep going.

A strong sense of purpose plays a key role in professional sports, too. Take the Oakland Athletics during the 2000s as an example. The organization's purpose was not only to be competitive with the best teams in Major League Baseball—organizations with deep pockets that fielded teams with the highest payrolls in the league—but to be competitive by following a different strategy in how it built its roster of players. The Oakland A's were a smaller market team, which meant they couldn't spend $200 million on a roster. The A's general manager, Billy Beane, knew this and recognized that he couldn't pay for star players who led the leagues in home runs, like the New York Yankees or Boston Red Sox did. Instead, he focused on identifying the key statistics that led to wins, like on-base percentage. Players who excelled in this statistic were generally undervalued by the rest of the league, only because those other teams overlooked the statistic's importance. That sense of purpose—of competing and winning by following a different (unproven) formula—was the thing that kept the Oakland Athletics focused on what must be done to succeed. The team made the playoffs after following this strategy in 2002, and even though they didn't win a championship, the team did set an American League record with 20 consecutive victories during the regular season.

James Kerr, in his book *Legacy*, spotlights New Zealand's All Blacks rugby team (named for their original black jerseys and knickerbockers) and showcases another way that purpose and meaning can play a pivotal role in sports. The team is constructed around a culture and a powerful legacy. Players on this team demand excellence from themselves and each other; they're led by a purpose to further that team legacy, living up to the expectations and the legacies of players who came before them and establishing an even stronger legacy for future players to adopt and expand upon. All Black players strive to be better on the field, plus they push one another to become better human beings off the field through community service. It all ties back to the concept of creating and furthering a lasting legacy.

Individual athletes, like weightlifter Mattie Rogers, also focus on their purpose, which manifests itself as the goals they want to achieve. "My why to get through hard days is knowing how much work I have put in to get to this point," she says, "And knowing that stopping or giving up would be throwing away so many days that I struggled through and came out on top even when I did not think I could. I know what I want to accomplish and I know I'm nowhere near that yet, so I try and take the hard times day by day and rep by rep and get as much out of myself as I can that day."

SELLING YOUR PURPOSES

With the rising popularity of social media, it's becoming easier to spot the "influencers" who are pushing products just to make a quick buck. In the nutrition and fitness world, these influencers are often scantily clad and pedaling the latest fat-loss supplements or detox teas. As the sales and promotional landscape continues to evolve, companies are finding that it's more important than ever to cultivate an authentic and honest relationship with the people who are essentially showcasing their products. When you have a true purpose—your "why"—you'll find it easier to relate to your customers, because those customers will recognize that your purpose is to create products that help people. In short, that authentic purpose will lead to greater success.

Human beings are emotional creatures. We are often guided first and most strongly by our emotions, as opposed to logic or reason. By sharing your (or your company's) purpose, you are also sharing with customers your story; the emotional ties to those stories can go a long way in helping people to understand your purpose and support it. As Simon Sinek points out, Apple's loyal customer base was first formed in 1984 following the brand's Super Bowl commercial, which implied that Apple's new and introductory personal computer would be unlike anything on the market. The tagline of the advertisement—"You'll see why 1984 won't be like 1984"— referenced George Orwell's dystopian novel to suggest that a person who bought an Apple computer would be an individualist, someone who made their own decisions and shaped the direction of their own lives. The commercial resonated with a lot of people and its emotional tie stuck.

Even today, people continue to buy Apple products because of the company's commitment and purpose to being different, instead of being driven by whether the products are better than those produced by a competitor.

In regards to my own company, Renaissance Periodization, our team members value our commitment to being an evidence-based company. They never promise easy results, they only promise that if you bring your work ethic, they will provide a plan to help you reach your fitness goals. The company also established the Renaissance Science Scholarship Fund at the University of Michigan in 2017. After I founded RP with my business partner Dr. Mike Israetel, we agreed that we wanted to give back to the school and its Kinesiology program that had given us our start. I believe that both these aspects of our business—a focus on evidence and helping others—have helped us to create our success. When you are true to your purpose, it no longer becomes a sales pitch. Instead, your purpose—once you share it with the public—naturally attracts people to what you are doing. I have never been particularly good at sales, but I've always worked hard, remained true to my commitment to help as many people as I can, and fostered a spirit of authenticity. Those attributes are what shaped RP's success.

THE RIGHT MOTIVATION

According to business author Daniel Pink, motivation is made up of three components: autonomy, mastery, and purpose.

We've already discussed autonomy and how the power to make your own choices is an important ingredient in the recipe for success. And it only makes sense that mastery—the acquisition or development of the skills necessary to complete tasks—is a factor of motivation, since you'll feel more compelled to set a new goal if you already have confidence in your ability to accomplish it. Not surprisingly, purpose is an integral piece of motivation, too; a great or desirable cause can keep you on track to put in the necessary work.

However, motivation is not constant—even for the most successful and committed professional athletes. Annie Thorisdottir has opened up about that very topic on Renaissance Periodiziation podcasts. "Obviously, I'm motivated," she says. "But nobody is motivated all of the time. We're so hooked on having to be motivated all of the time. We don't have to. It's perfectly fine to have these moments where you're not. My thing is just knowing why I'm doing the things that I'm doing. I know why I go to the gym. I have my reasons for wanting to get better. . . . . As long as I know my *why*, it's not a question of whether I'm going to go or not. I am going to go whether I'm motivated or I'm not motivated, whether I feel like it or I don't feel like it. I'm going to go to the gym. I'm going to put in my best effort of that day and that is how I know that I'm doing absolutely everything in my power to become the best version of myself."

The concept of a greater sense of purpose defines some of the most recognizable corporations. As Jim Collins reveals in his book *Good to Great*, the executive team behind Walmart has always been fanatical about selling goods at the lowest possible prices. The company's motto—"We save people money so they can live better"—reflects this purpose, and it was something that the company's founder, Sam Walton, stressed from the beginning. In fact, some corporate decisions, like streamlining Walmart headquarters of any plush amenities, were made specifically so that the company could adhere to its larger purpose.

The Zappos shoe brand provides another great example, which the company's former CEO, Tony Hsieh, details in his book *Delivering Happiness*. According to Hsieh, he constructed a corporate culture that made his employees excited to come to work, and that spilled over into the work that they performed. Because they enjoyed being at work, Zappos employees were committed to instilling a similar level of happiness in the customers who were purchasing shoes on the company's website. Exceptional customer service was always Hsieh's number one goal, and by keeping that purpose in mind, he was able to take the necessary steps to accomplish it.

A HIGHER CALLING – NAVY SEALS

To subject yourself to the type of training that is needed to become an elite Special Forces operative requires a higher calling. I've read as many books about the Navy SEALs as I can, and a prevailing theme across all of those books is the call to service that is required to be a Navy SEAL. The soldiers who graduate to that rank have a higher sense of purpose, and that purpose provides them with the necessary motivation to fight with and for their brothers in arms as they serve their country. As Roy F. Baumeister and John Tierney explain in *Willpower: Rediscovering the Greatest Human Strength*, that focus on a purpose bigger than your own is what allows you to push yourself further. It's at the core of what allows the Navy SEALs to accomplish their missions. In fact, the Navy SEALs prove that philosopher Friedrich Nietzsche was right. "He who has a why to live," Nietzsche said, "can bear almost any how."

Conversations that I've had with friends of mine who are Navy SEALs reinforce this belief. That higher sense of purpose, they've told me, allows them to endure things that exceed most people's limits. One Navy SEAL, who grew up as an only child, connected with his teammates as brothers, and that sense of brotherhood became his higher purpose. "Having the closest thing to a brother I have ever known," he says, "and not wanting to disappoint them or let them down was what kept me going."

After learning about the Navy SEAL culture, which supports a higher purpose of brotherhood and accountability, it becomes easier to understand how those elite operatives can successfully complete such dangerous and important missions. "We're in this business because we believe in it—because of who we are," says former Navy SEAL Dick Couch in his book *The Warrior Elite*. "It is the desire to belong to an elite group—to become a warrior. Those who succeed have high expectations of themselves, and they want to associate with others who share those expectations."

TOO MUCH PURPOSE

The flipside of purpose is having too much: being so committed to a purpose that you lose the ability to rationally analyze the world around you. As way of example, let me introduce a throwback to the early 1970s—the creation of Atari. Nolan Bushnell founded Atari in 1972 and, in doing so, he laid the groundwork for modern-day video games. Bushnell had a passion and a commitment to science fiction and he loved technology. These passions served him well; Atari games like Asteroids were a smash hit. After Atari was acquired, however, Bushnell became too consumed by his love affair with technology and his desire to pave the way for the future. Eventually, he was forced out of Atari, so he tried to make it on his own. He attempted to start numerous other bootstrapped tech companies, yet with every opportunity his futuristic vision got the best of him. He invested himself in so many different avenues that none of them sustained success after Atari. Ultimately, Bushnell was deemed to be too far ahead of his time, which prevented the necessary groundwork from being laid to take his post-Atari business enterprises mainstream.

Bushnell's story is a cautionary tale of the risks that can come from being too consumed with your greater purpose. In Bushnell's case, he was focused on too many sci-fi projects. You should be deeply passionate about your work, but you should also be able to focus on your efforts in the here and now. There is a fine line to walk in this regard. Ultimately, you should find your passion and harness your energy toward a goal, but you must not lose sight of the work that must be done today to reach that goal. Your focus must remain on the work that you do today—but use your passion and your greater purpose as the compass to lead you in the right direction.

PURPOSE ROOTED IN REAL LIFE

Many successful businesspeople and well-known entrepreneurs have carefully molded their purpose around a specific vision for what they want to create, be it a product or an enterprise. But your purpose doesn't have to be crafted in a similar manner. In fact, your purpose may not be a vision of business success at all. In some cases, you may find that your purpose is developed around the important personal relationships in your life.

Nita Strauss follows a dual purpose, one inspired by

those whom she loves and one directed toward those who have questioned her abilities. Her purpose is to make her family and friends proud since, as she acknowledges, they "believed in me and expected the best from me when I didn't believe in myself." However, she also reveals that she works hard "to prove any doubters in my field wrong."

Finding purpose and meaning through a personal relationship can be a powerful guide as you establish a career or strive for excellence. Just ask Erik Bakich, the head coach of the University of Michigan baseball team, who implements RP principles into his players' training regimens. He brought his team to the finals of the College World Series in 2019 and subsequently earned NCAA Coach of the Year honors. "I made a promise to my dying college coach before he passed away to continue his inspiration and his legacy," he says. "There is no amount of money I would trade for the experience and relationships made in college, and I want all players I get the opportunity to coach to have the same experience. That's the 'why' for my chosen coaching profession."

As Coach Bakich reveals, when your 'why' is large enough, it can supersede the allure of lucrative paychecks. A true purpose will be far more motivating than any amount of money. When you have a meaning like that, you will be far more likely to stay on the right path and remain dedicated to your goals and your overall mission.

Whatever your passion or career may be, a clearly defined sense of purpose can be your guiding star through the setbacks along the way. If your guiding star is bright enough, you will likely attract others to join you, and through that mutual collaboration you will increase your odds of significant success.

Yet, even with a resolute work ethic, self-direction, a positive mindset, plenty of discipline, and clarity of purpose, you will find that at times the going will be tough. There will be setbacks and challenges. You need a strong and meaningful purpose to follow and to focus on because during your journey you will fail. Failure is so common, in fact, that you should expect to fail along the way. And while we can't avoid failure, how we choose to respond to it will make a world of difference.

PUTTING IT INTO PRACTICE

Make a list of your core values—personal and/or professional—and place them somewhere you'll see them frequently. Many days you won't need a reminder of why you're putting in the work or what specifically you're working for, but there will be times when you'll grow frustrated, overwhelmed, or discouraged. On those days, this reminder will provide a necessary boost of morale to overcome any challenges that have temporarily gotten the better of you.

CHAPTER 6

FAILURE

" —
| There is no such thing as failure.
Failure is just life trying to move
us in another direction."

—OPRAH WINFREY

I KNOW WHAT YOU MUST BE THINKING. Why is there an entire chapter dedicated to failure in a book that is intended to provide readers with a roadmap to success? The short answer is this: as you pursue your goals you will occasionally be met by failure. It's almost inevitable that your journey will include moments of failure at one time or another. We are all human. We're not infallible. Mistakes happen and failures occur, but how you respond to those failures can dictate whether or not you eventually find success. It takes a special person to take failure on the chin, check their ego at the door, and to learn from their mistakes. But oftentimes that is what's required to be successful.

Human beings learn best from trial and error. We make mistakes but we figure out how to correct them, and we do this from a very young age. A toddler who is learning to walk will stumble and fall, but they'll pick themselves up and keep trying. In time, they'll be walking with steadiness. And they'll soon learn to run by following this same process. It is part of the human condition to learn from mistakes. "Your child needs practice failing," Amy Morin writes in her book, *13 Things Mentally Strong Parents Don't Do*, "so he can learn to rebound."

Yet, when we get older, we go to school and we're taught that making mistakes is bad, that mistakes are a sign of weakness or a mark of inferiority. We lose points on tests for the mistakes that we make, and after at least a dozen years of schooling, we're conditioned to equate mistakes with poor performance. Not surprisingly, people become scared of failure; they certainly don't believe that failure begets success.

However, to make mistakes is distinctly human, as Kathryn Schulz explains in *Being Wrong: Adventures in the Margin of Error*. According to Schulz, human beings have the advantage of a strong belief system, and if we believe that errors and mistakes are inevitable, we'll be much better off. Knowing that we are not infallible will help us make better choices. Rather than always fighting to be right, we should embrace learning from the mistakes and the errors that we'll almost certainly make along the way.

This idea is hardly new. People have learned from their failures for thousands of years. Take the 21-year reign of Genghis Khan, who founded the Mongol Empire, as way of example. Jack Weatherford documents in his book *Genghis Khan and the Making of the Modern World* that the emperor rose to power and created an empire without any formal education or divine enlightenment. "His success," writes Weatherford, "was derived from a persistent cycle of pragmatic learning, experimental adaptation and constant revision driven by his uniquely disciplined and focused will."

MINDSET

Being able to adapt, to grow, and to change based on the results of our actions is paramount. Charles Darwin proved this through his discovery and subsequent study of evolution. It is not the strongest species that survive, nor the most intelligent, Darwin observed. Instead, the ones most responsive to change are the ones that succeed. This concept of adaptation reflects back on the notion that a growth mindset is more valuable than one that is fixed. If you have a growth mindset, you see failure and obstacles as ways to learn and expand. But if you have a fixed mindset, even the thought of failure is terrifying.

Anyone who doubts the validity of this association only needs to consider the career of one of the most successful professional athletes of all time. "I've missed more than 9,000 shots in my career," Michael Jordan once acknowledged. "I have lost almost 300 games. Twenty-six times, I have been trusted to take the game-winning shot and missed. I have failed over and over and over again in my life. And that is why I succeed."

Can you imagine the greatest basketball player of all time shying away from taking the game-winning shot because he was afraid of failure? With that mindset, he would never become the best of all time. No one likes to fail, of course, and psychologists have even proven that people have a strong aversion to failure (read *Thinking, Fast and Slow* by Daniel Kahneman for more info). But the important thing is to first acknowledge that failure might—and often will—occur, and then commit yourself to the task with all your effort anyway. Michael Jordan was successful in part because of his ability, but also because he adopted the right mindset and took the right approach to possible failure.

Those who have a growth mindset, who embrace new challenges and the setbacks that come with them, will learn more and improve more than those who are intimidated by the possibility of failure. In fact, the most successful people often view failure as a positive. They recognize that each failure is a small step toward eventual success. "I have not failed," Thomas Edison famously declared when asked about his journey to invent the lightbulb, "I have just found 10,000 ways that don't work." That is the type of mindset that overcomes setbacks and perseveres when failures do occur.

Perfection may be the goal, but it shouldn't be your expectation. Dieting provides an ideal example. Someone who follows a three-month diet plan, which allows them to have five smaller meals per day, will be faced with 450 opportunities to mess up. The people who achieve the best results when dieting, based on my observations (and also data from the RP Diet App), typically adhere to their macro or caloric counts 85 to 90 percent of the time. That means you can be less-than-perfect on 50 of those 450 total meals and the odds will still be in your favor to achieve great results.

It's important to note, however, that the people who slip up on one meal during a day don't let that mistake spiral out of control. If they did, mistakes during one meal would multiply into mistakes made for every subsequent meal that day. Soon, that negative momentum carries over into multiple days and then, before you know it, you've lost an entire week . . . sometimes even a month. At that point, with your momentum gone, it's easy to throw in the towel. Kelly McGonigal, in her book *The Willpower Instinct*, refers to this as the "what-the-hell effect." The basic idea is that general consistency is more powerful than attempting to be perfect.

Tim Grover, one of the top trainers in professional basketball, has worked with Hall of Famers like Michael Jordan and Kobe Bryant. In his book *Relentless,* Grover describes those athletes as cleaners. Grover explains the cleaners' attitude like this: "You can't control or anticipate every obstacle that might block your path. You can only control your response, and your ability to navigate the unpredictable." When you pair that type of stoicism with a growth mindset, suddenly, challenges and failures don't seem so upsetting. If you can adopt that way of thinking, you will see obstacles as tools, simple pieces of information that will help you to shape your new path.

Professional sports provide proof that occasional failure doesn't prevent success. Championship teams in the NBA, for example, lose around 20 games during the regular season each year—even more if you count the playoffs. Or think about it this way: a Major League Baseball player who carries a .300 batting average for his career is almost guaranteed to be voted into the Hall of Fame. That means that the greatest players in history failed more than two-thirds of the time that they stepped up to the plate.

Professional sports also teach us that initial failures can be overcome and the highest level of success still achieved. Bill Walsh, who coached the San Francisco 49ers to three Super Bowl championships during the 1980s, nearly stepped down as head coach early in his career after two losing seasons. During the first two years that Walsh served as head coach, his team won only eight games and lost twenty-four. But Walsh learned from his mistakes during those first two seasons; in 1981, he led the 49ers to their first Super Bowl championship and subsequently earned Coach of the Year honors.

Even super forecasters (for sports bets and other projections) adopt this type of mindset. These professionals, who are known to successfully predict future outcomes more than the so-called experts, are always learning, growing, and keeping an open mind. They take new evidence as it comes to them and modify their predictions as necessary. They also almost never speak in absolutes. Instead, they refer to percentage likelihood. If they feel that an event is probable, they might declare that they are 70 or 80 percent confident. They understand that even successful individuals are wrong a lot of the time.

OBSTACLES ARE OPPORTUNITIES

Successful individuals have a habit of seeing failures or challenges as an opportunity to better themselves. Even in times of panic or crisis, those individuals generally remain calmer, use logic and reason, don't let their emotions get in the way, and consider how they can leverage the challenge to improve themselves or their situation. During a lecture to the U.S. Naval Academy, Dan Luna, a retired U.S. Navy veteran and retired Navy SEAL summed that up in a very succinct way. "Obstacles are opportunities," he told the audience.

This notion that obstacles, failures, and crises can be beneficial in the business world is an idea supported by Andy Grove, the former CEO of Intel. "Bad companies are destroyed by crisis," he explains. "Good companies survive them. Great companies are improved by them." To improve during difficult times, you must first identify your areas of weakness and then devote time and resources to them. Even during challenging times, you can choose where you focus your time, energy, money, and other resources. Many situations are just that—situations. In most cases they're neither inherently good nor bad; it's up to us to determine that based on how we perceive them. Successful individuals play the hand that they have been dealt and figure out a way to work with what they have. If you choose to focus on self-pity, you'll end up ruminating on the hardships in front of you rather than troubleshooting a way out of the hard times you are currently in.

Oftentimes, the obstacles that you encounter will reveal a distinct, slightly different path than the one you were originally on; but that new path is the one that will lead to success, or at least get you closer to it. Contemporary author Ryan Holiday emphasizes this point in his book *The Obstacle Is the Way*, in which he explains that the challenge that stands in your path today will eventually become the way for you to move forward. This perception is borrowed from Roman emperor Marcus Aurelius, who declared during his reign from 161 to 180 AD: "The impediment to action advances action. What stands in the way becomes the way."

Whatever you encounter or are presented with, make the choice to perceive it as a positive. Lessons can be learned from everything. Being passed over for a promotion at work will reveal to you the things that you need to work on. A bad test grade in school will make you realize that you must study harder and also make changes to your study habits or routine. If you fail a lift at the gym, you'll know that you need to improve your nutrition, devote more time to recovery, or alter your workout program altogether. That old proverb "whatever doesn't kill you makes you stronger" is generally true.

This is the mindset that I brought to Lori's cancer diagnosis in early 2020, and it was a mindset that I was able to maintain through months of quarantining during the coronavirus pandemic that followed. Yes, I was stuck at home, but I decided that was good. It gave me time to solidify my routines and habits. I had an opportunity to homeschool my kids and to help them with their education. It provided me an opportunity to write this book. No matter how bad the situation seemed, I was determined to not consider myself a victim of those circumstances. Instead, I was going to come out of it all better than ever, and my kids were going to be smarter when they returned to school and more skilled when they went back to their Brazilian jiujitsu classes.

When things seem dire, the easy road is accepting a victim's role. Don't take it. Instead, take control of your mindset and focus on the things that you can control. Be disciplined in your implementation of a new, positive attitude.

FAILURE IS INEVITABLE

The world that we live in is chaotic and unpredictable. The coronavirus pandemic certainly proved that. Even the world's best super forecasters are wrong the majority of the time. What does all of this mean for those of us who aren't exceptionally skilled at predicting the future? It means we are bound to be wrong a lot of the time. Even some of the world's greatest leaders—Alexander the Great, Napoleon Bonaparte, and Winston Churchill—all made major mistakes during their lives and during their periods of command. Because the world we live in is often crazy and unpredictable, the best way to learn is simply through trial and error. That's the message that author Tim Harford shares in his book *Adapt: Why Success Always Starts with Failure.*

Think of your ideas as different species. Then consider what we now know about natural selection and evolution. Survival of the fittest means that many of your ideas are going to fail. But it also means that the best ideas and the best adaptations of failed ideas will rise to the top. Those ideas and adaptations represent success, or at least the pathway to it. When marketing executives create social media campaigns, for example, they typically start by selecting 10 to 20 images to use, but they anticipate that the majority of those images won't be effective. They're only looking for a few standouts that make an impact, which will guide them toward understanding what visuals to use going forward.

Just remember, this process of change and adaptation never stops. The moment you think you can stop is likely the moment that your competition will pass you by.

If you want to improve, you must be open to feedback. Peter Palchinsky, a brilliant engineer who worked for the now-defunct Soviet Union, conceived of three principles related to failure and adaptation, which Harford outlines in his aforementioned book. Those three principles are:

1. Seek out new ideas and try new things.
2. Make your first attempts small when you can, so you can survive if they don't succeed.
3. Seek out feedback and learn from your mistakes.

These may seem simple and they may sound like common sense. But when you factor in ego and other human biases, these mantras are anything but simple. If you wish to be successful, you must always keep an open mind and you must be tolerable to new ideas and honest feedback.

Failure to do those things will likely lead to failure overall.

If you're still not convinced, read *Why Smart Executives Fail: And What You Can Learn from Their Mistakes* by Sydney Finkelstein. As the author explains, very smart and highly accomplished individuals fail—and so do the organizations that they run—precisely because their egos get in the way. They fail to take action when presented with evidence that contradicts their previously held beliefs, and they purposefully avoid seeking out advice and perspectives that may challenge their views. In short, they are stubborn and believe that their views are always correct.

Starting out small is something that many people struggle with, simply because they're enthusiastic to get started and they've been conditioned to believe that the only way to succeed is to do everything that they can. Yes, they'll eventually need to put in all of their effort, but it's best to ramp up to that, especially if you have no prior experience in what you are attempting and therefore no knowledge that it's the right approach to take. If you experiment on large-scale projects that take up most of your time and resources, you are likely setting yourself up for failure that will be too great to recover from.

FEEDBACK & LEARNING

While you can learn from failure at any time, there are points along your journey to success when failure can be more beneficial. In particular, failure that occurs quickly—and in the beginning—can often be a better teaching mechanism than failure that occurs over a longer period of time. "Your first try will be wrong," says Aza Raskin, the creative lead at Mozilla Corporation, which developed the Firefox internet browser. "Budget and design for it."

Think of golf, specifically putting. Obviously, the goal is to get the ball into the hole in as few strokes as possible. But think of how much more difficult it would be to make a putt if you couldn't see how the ball rolled after you hit it. Now imagine that you can suddenly see what the ball does. You can see how quickly or slowly it rolls, whether it turns to the right or the left, or not at all. Your next putt becomes much easier. Instant feedback like that can have a similar effect in business. Immediate (or quick) results allow you to make better decisions earlier in the process. As authors Richard Thaler and Cass Sunstein write in their book *Nudge*: "Learning is most likely if people get immediate, clear feedback after each try."

In particular, the human brain needs immediate feedback to solve problems. It takes a lot for human beings to deviate from homeostasis, so if we don't receive clear direction or guidance based on our current actions, we're likely to continuing acting in the same manner that we always have. This is known as the status quo bias. When tasked with having to make a choice, people are generally more inclined to hit the easy button.

Cognitive dissonance is another bias that can interfere with our ability to properly respond to failure. After making a mistake or failing in some way, your initial response may include thoughts like, "I'm a failure." But in the next instant, you may think, "I made a mistake. Now I need to move on and correct it." Those two thoughts are at conflict with one another, and the challenge is to condition yourself to hold onto the second thought and to dismiss the first. Ego and general stubbornness can play a role in making this more difficult than it seems. As Daniel Kahneman explains in *Thinking, Fast and Slow*, human beings are averse to loss, which means we are more likely to hold onto a bad idea (or one that has failed) thinking that we can turn things around. Doing so prevents us from acknowledging that we failed. But remember that failure is sometimes necessary to achieve success.

You must also be careful of another bias: hedonic editing, which Harford outlines in *Adapt: Why Success Always Starts with Failure*. This is the desire to want to merge the good with the bad. For example, if you make two financial investments and one gains $5,000 but the other loses $2,500, you may say that you still came out ahead, that you're up $2,500. This lessens the emotional impact of the failure, but it also makes it harder to learn the proper lessons and to improve from the mistakes that led to that failure. Businesses can make this mistake as well, especially those that create multiple products or variations of the same product. If they group all of those products together into a single sales figure, business owners will have difficulty analyzing the ones that aren't delivering results, since their numbers will be skewed by the ones that are selling. I have trained my team at RP to pay close attention to the company products that add minimal value. This allows us to devote more resources to the ones that are providing the best returns.

ITERATE

Those who have experience with start-up businesses are likely to know the term MVP. It stands for Minimum Viable Product. As explained by Eric Ries in the book *The*

Lean Startup, an MVP is a product that you may not be 100 percent happy with, but that allows you to validate your hypotheses. It is likely low risk and it should represent a minimal amount of financial investment. The purpose of an MVP is to gather feedback from consumers. You may know that there are areas in which you can improve the product and that there are challenges to overcome, but an MVP allows you to test your ideas and, more importantly, to iterate and improve based on the feedback that you receive.

To continually iterate is to acknowledge that what you're doing now is better than what you did before. But, it also comes with the understanding that what you're doing now won't be as good as what you are likely to do in the future. You want to embrace sending your ideas out in the world for that real-life feedback. Receiving that feedback and subsequently iterating based on what you learn is a tried-and-true formula for positive achievements. "The real measure of success," Thomas Edison once said, "is the number of experiments that can be crowded into twenty-four hours."

At RP, we followed this strategy by unveiling digital diet templates in early 2015 that were clunky Excel files. They didn't look like much, but they delivered great results. We released them in that rough-around-the-edges format to make sure that the general product concept was one that our potential customers would buy and use. We received great feedback—and our clients achieved exceptional results—so we iterated in 2016, improving the original formulas to produce even better results. Still, the templates weren't polished in their appearance. In 2017, we iterated again, this time to improve the look and feel of the product, but even as we did that, we knew that we would soon replace those templates with a dynamic and interactive option offered through the RP Diet App, which we were building based on all of the user feedback we had received to that point. Today, we continue to iterate along the way through constant software development.

Consider the social media platform Facebook. For more than 15 years, Facebook has refined its approach and evolved its offerings based on data that it has gathered from the feedback provided by millions of its members. Similarly, Gmail (email by Google) for years was branded as "beta," even though millions of users had already signed on to use it.

Perhaps the best example of iteration is Apple's iPhone. Today, the smartphone can do seemingly everything under the sun, but remarkably, the first generation of the phone was lacking options as basic as a "copy" function. That goes to show how much Apple has committed to iteration and it helps to explain why and how the company has become so successful. If you wait until your product is perfect, you may miss the chance to capitalize on what you've created. But if you take a chance and roll out something that still has the potential to be better, you can gather invaluable feedback to help you improve it.

While recording a podcast, I was once asked where I thought RP would be five years in the future. My answer was only that it would be remarkably better than what it was at that time. I knew that we would commit ourselves to constantly improving little by little. That is how you become successful. You constantly seek the little improvements and you stay on that path. The incremental changes compound themselves over time. You might not even realize that progress is being made on a daily basis, but over time "little by little" eventually becomes a lot and the changes can be drastic.

CULTURE

Creating a culture at work that supports learning and improvement via feedback—in other words, a culture that acknowledges that failures are part of the process—can enhance businesses' ultimate success. It also stands to reason that a culture dictated by indignant leaders who berate those who have made mistakes can be counterproductive. In such a scenario, it's not unreasonable to imagine people trying to hide or cover up for mistakes if the consequences of making them are so severe.

That being said, exceptions should be made after severe mistakes, ones that jeopardize safety or lead to sizeable losses in revenue. But even in those cases, a successful leader will own the mistakes of his or her colleagues and will look to make procedural changes or fix training protocols to ensure those mistakes aren't made again. In their book *In Search of Excellence*, Tom Peters and Robert Waterman write: "Tolerance for failure is a very specific part of the excellent company culture—and that lesson comes directly from the top. Champions have to make lots of tries and consequently suffer some failures or the organization won't learn."

More than 20 years after that book's publication, successful executives still acknowledge this to be true. "I make mistakes all the time and talk about them openly with people up and down our hierarchy," said Dave Finocchio, the former CEO of Bleacher Report. "It fosters a culture where people should feel comfortable critiquing themselves honestly."

The U.S. Air Force serves as a great example of the successes that can come from understanding that mistakes happen and that accomplishments are created by the lessons learned from those mistakes. As Anders Ericsson and Robert Pool chronicle in *Peak: Secrets from the New Science of Expertise*, the U.S. Air Force created its Top Gun program to remedy its struggles in air combat during the Vietnam War. Pilots in the program would engage in training combat scenarios with their instructors, then conduct "postmortem" analyses to go over why specific decisions were made and key factors or details that were missed. That immediate feedback allowed those pilots to make positive strides right away. Just how successful has the program been? The numbers tell the story. During the Vietnam War in the late 1960s, two enemy aircraft were shot down for every one U.S. fighter jet that was shot down. By the end of the Persian Gulf War in 1991, however, American pilots were shooting down more than 30 enemy fighter jets for every one U.S. aircraft that was shot down.

TOO MUCH FAILURE

It's certainly clear by now that failure can lead to success, but like everything in life, too much of any one thing can be problematic. When it comes to failure, that can take the form of too many small failures—they do add up over time—or too much failure all in one fell swoop. Failures can be helpful, so long as lessons are learned from them. When those lessons aren't realized—usually because too much ego is involved—the failures will begin to add up, some-times repeating themselves. At that point, you and your venture could be doomed.

A big component to success is being able to handle the dichotomy of too much and too little ego. Those who are successful tend to have an ego, but they use it to funnel themselves in the right direction. Their ego drives them to be successful; it fuels their hard work and discipline, but it does not overcome them. It does not blind them to learning from their own mistakes and being able to pivot accordingly. You must be able to balance that dichotomy, and as you mature it should get easier to spot when things cross the line. Aim to be self-aware and honest with your-self. Having a good team or support system in place can go a long way in helping with this, since those teammates will let you know when you begin to cross the line and when your ego is too active in the decision-making process.

It isn't always easy to make the right choices or deci-sions. A study of U.S. judges presiding over parole hearings, as outlined in Roy Baumeister and John Tierney's *Will-power: Rediscovering the Greatest Human Strength*, pro-vides necessary proof. According to the study, judges were more lenient or more generous with granting parole when they were well-rested or immediately after they had eaten lunch. Conversely, they were less lenient as they grew tired or hungry. There's a takeaway from this study that can help everyone. If you're forced to make a tough decision, aim to do it in the morning, when you're well rested, or shortly after you've eaten, when your blood sugar (and energy level) is at its highest. Just be careful of a scenario in which many difficult choices must be made at the same time. In those circumstances, it's not uncommon for decision-makers to fall into the status quo bias, especially as they begin to feel mentally taxed from the difficult decisions that they've already had to make.

REAL WORLD VIEW

Failure is simply a part of life. It's also a part of most great success stories. Any successful person's biography will be strewn with stories about hardships, mistakes, and failures. Take *Shoe Dog* by Phil Knight, which provides an insider's glimpse at how Nike was created. Regularly throughout the book—seemingly at least once in each chapter—the reader learns that for quite a long while the company was hanging on by a thread. Mistakes were made and friendships were lost. Yet, in the end, Nike and its "Just Do It" slogan are prevalent throughout sports all around the world.

There are plenty of other stories that reveal the early-career failures of today's well known celebrities or successful artists. Stephen King's first book idea was rejected more than 30 times. At one point in her life J.K. Rowling (creator of Harry Potter) was a single mother on government assistance. Even Walt Disney was once deemed to "lack imagination." We all know how Disney rebounded from that evaluation.

The key is not avoiding mistakes altogether or shying away from failure. Instead, what makes people successful is their ability to weather the storm with the right mindset. "I understand they happen, and they are to be expected," Navy SEAL Dan Luna says of mistakes. "Often, I will separate it logically and emotionally to examine the setback or mistake."

"It's always easier to blame others or external factors when something doesn't go the way you want it," adds Annie Thorisdottir. "However, it's crucial to look inwards first, see if something that you are in control of could have altered the outcome of the situation, and devise a plan on how to make sure this does not repeat itself in the future."

Success does not happen overnight. Instead, it is cultivated by the repetition of high-level effort and redirection when failure occurs. At the end of the day, the act of success requires a whole lot of work—work that is done in an uncertain, always-changing environment, and work that is done without any guarantee of accomplishment. In fact, that work only guarantees at least some, occasional failure.

This path can become exhausting, and if you're going to travel down it long enough to see eventual success, you'll need ways to shed this fatigue and to recharge your pursuit.

PUTTING IT INTO PRACTICE

Make a list of your three biggest failures to date and what, in hindsight, you might have done differently. This exercise will help train your mind to connect mistakes or failures with the lessons that can be gleaned from them. You can then use the information that you obtain from that analysis to set new goals and sub-goals that will keep you motivated.

CHAPTER 7

—

RECHARGE

" —
Energy, not time, is the fundamental
currency of high performance."

—JIM LOEHR

BEING SUCCESSFUL IS NOT EASY. Moreover, it can be draining. Even a person who enjoys that struggle and enjoys working exceptionally hard toward a specific goal can push too hard for too long and burn out. Fortunately, there are steps that can (and should) be taken to prevent this. First, acknowledge your limits and the need to recharge. Anyone who's looking to achieve success must realize that keeping their foot on the gas pedal will eventually leave their tank empty. In the quest for success, the notion of burning the candle from both ends is a legitimate risk. By taking the proper steps to recharge yourself, you can avoid the pitfalls of burnout.

RECHARGING PHYSICALLY THROUGH NUTRITION

Nutrition is a fundamental key to recharging. If you want to perform at your best, you need to dial in your nutrition habits. A Ferrari owner would never fuel up with regular unleaded gasoline. They'd only select super premium at the pumps, knowing that their sports car won't perform the way it should at 200-mile-per-hour speeds if its gas tank is full of low-quality fuel. Your body and mind work the same way.

A well-balanced diet is the goal. Achieving that requires an understanding of six nutritional priorities for healthy eating. (For a deeper dive into performance nutrition, refer to *The Renaissance Diet 2.0*).

Nutritional Priority #1 – Calorie Balance: One key to being successful is longevity. Very few people become successful overnight. The longer you are alive, the better your chances of finding success. Calorie balance plays the biggest role in your nutritional strides for better longevity, since it has the largest impact on your weight. You definitely don't want to overeat, which puts you in a caloric surplus, but you don't want to under-eat, either. As doctors Mike Israetel, Jen Case, and Trevor Pfaendtner explain in *Understanding Healthy Eating: A Science-Based Guide to How Your Diet Affects Your Health*, maintaining a healthy bodyweight is a critical step in establishing longevity and boosting your overall health.

For evidence, look at offensive and defensive linemen in the NFL. They know that to be the best and to perform at an elite level, they need to be a certain size. However, once they retire, most of those linemen look to lose a significant amount of weight. They know that they can't continue to be 300-plus pounds and expect to live long and healthy lives.

Nutritional Priority #2 – Food Quality: The best way to maintain a healthy bodyweight while consuming fewer calories is by eating high-quality foods. If you focus your diet only on the food choices outlined in the Brain Food section of Chapter 3, you'll find it almost impossible to overeat. This means consuming mostly lean proteins, fruits/vegetables, healthy fats, and healthy carbs like whole grains. If you need help controlling your caloric intake, focus on eating less junk food. By eliminating fast food and regular soda (some diet soda is ok), you will make it easier on yourself to lower your calories, which will get you to a healthier bodyweight.

Nutritional Priority #3 – Macronutrients: When you eat for health, first and foremost you must focus on the amount of protein in your diet. Most people don't eat enough protein, but this is easily corrected. As long as you don't have any pre-existing medical conditions, eating more protein than you need is much less of a problem than not eating enough of it. In fact, increasing your protein intake will likely help you to retain more lean tissue while shedding unwanted body fat. And because protein is satiating, eating more of it will leave you feeling less hungry throughout the day. Beyond that, so long as you're consuming a healthy number of calories each day, it generally doesn't matter how many total grams of carbohydrates or grams of fat you are eating. In other words, if you control your caloric intake and you consume enough protein, your split between carbohydrates and fats matters much less. (The opposite is true if you are eating for optimal body composition. But in this scenario, we're only outlining the best ways to eat for general health.)

Nutritional Priority #4 – Nutrient Timing: When you're

eating for health, the timing of when you eat barely mat-ters. Eating a regimented diet of high-quality foods and sticking to a healthy caloric intake each day are the most important steps. In other words, eating two or three larger meals a day is no better or worse than choosing to eat five or six smaller meals. This is great news for entrepreneurs and busy individuals, as it provides more flexibility for your meal schedule.

Nutritional Priority #5 – Hydration: While obesity is a legitimate concern in the United States, dehydration is not. If you're making sure to drink when you feel thirsty, you're generally on the right track. But a good way to gauge your level of hydration is to monitor the color of your urine. If it's mostly clear, you're drinking enough fluids throughout the day. (Please note: those who are training for and competing in athletic or endurance events will require a more rigorous review of their hydration.)

Nutritional Priority #6 – Supplements: Too many peo-ple think that supplements are magical pills that will boost their training or weight loss results or their chances of suc-cess. They're not. If you eat a well-balanced diet, you gen-erally don't need to take any supplements whatsoever. But because we live busy lives, it's not always possible to eat well-balanced meals all the time. In those instances, sup-plementing with a basic multivitamin and fish oil can fill in the holes. They can act as an insurance policy if you do have lapses in your diet from time to time. Other items, like protein powders, protein bars, or ready-to-drink shakes are worthy supplement options, too. They're not mandatory, of course, but their added convenience can be a blessing for many of us living busy lives.

The most important lesson about nutrition for general health—and as a recharge—is to stick to the fundamentals. Claims that promise the world or seem like a quick and easy fix should be met with skepticism, since there's no evidence to support that those magic cures actually work. For more detailed insight into nutrition for general health, read the aforementioned book *Understanding Healthy Eating*. Just remember, consistently sticking to a solid nutrition plan is what matters most.

RECHARGING PHYSICALLY THROUGH EXERCISE

The same basic principles of good nutrition also apply to exercise. Magical exercises that boost your productivity or decrease that "stubborn belly fat," like all those television commercials and magazine advertisements promise, simply do not exist. What does provide results, however, is long-term consistency and dedication to regular exercise. Finding an activity that you enjoy can go a long way toward making those two things very attainable.

Strength and resistance training with weights has been shown to offer many health benefits, including reduced likelihood of osteoporosis and increased overall quality of life in a person's later years. And, best of all, effective, life-changing exercise doesn't require extensive time commitments. A few short sessions per week might be all that is necessary to improve your general health. You don't need fancy equipment or exercises either. Just stick to basic compound movements like squats, lunges, presses, and rows. Even better, convince a buddy to join you or join a class. That will provide some extra accountability, which will improve your chances of sticking with it.

Through exercise—especially exercise that pushes you outside of your comfort zone—you will not only strengthen your body, you'll condition and strengthen your mind. You'll improve your mental toughness by routinely working through situations where you feel uncomfortable. And when you combine that exercise with a healthy diet and good eating habits, you'll be taking the necessary steps to recharge. Stephen Covey, who wrote *The 7 Habits of Highly Effective People*, likens these actions to sharpening a saw. He reminds us that to perform at our best, we must take care of ourselves physically. Exercise and nutrition are two key components of that.

RECHARGING MENTALLY

Many of the self-improvement books dedicated to will-power and self-control tout the importance and the power of mindfulness and meditation. If the thought of meditation makes you roll your eyes, you're not alone. For the longest time I took a similar stance on the significance of meditation. But in all my reading on the general topic of self-improvement, I continued to discover that meditation plays an important part in the lives of many successful individuals. Eventually, I decided that I needed to give it an honest try for myself.

As I discovered, meditation is a great tool for reducing the amount of stress in your life. Sitting quietly and just being aware helps you to become more in tune with your thoughts and emotions. When you consistently practice mindfulness, you gain the ability to slow things down. That provides clarity and minimizes the impact that our emotions can have on the decisions that we make. Meditation can help people avoid the common pitfalls of cognitive biases. In fact, mediation has even been said to help increase creativity and the brain's efficiency.

Plenty of formal evidence exists to support the practice of meditation. We should all take time out of our days to be mindful. That doesn't necessarily mean that you have to meditate in a formal way. If you're skeptical about meditation, just do something that allows time for quiet reflection.

If the idea of structured meditation—or even quiet mindfulness—doesn't excite you, consider keeping a journal and writing down key thoughts or ideas that you have each day. In fact, Martin Seligman, in his book *Flourish: A Visionary New Understanding of Happiness and Well-being*, suggests journaling three blessings on a daily basis. When you focus on things for which you are grateful, you find that you gain a better appreciation for life in general. Gratitude is linked to a greater sense of well-being, and that improved state of being can improve overall performance.

During the quarantine period that we all lived through in 2020, I took a similar approach. Sure, I could have dwelled on the negative aspects of it all, thinking that I was stuck at home. Instead, I chose to be thankful and to cultivate feelings of gratitude. In my case, the quarantine provided me more time to spend with my family and more time to dedicate to my health. I made a point to be grateful and thankful that Amazon deliveries kept a steady stream of new books arriving on my front doorstep, and that meal-prep companies like Trifecta Nutrition could deliver exactly what I needed for food so that I only went to the grocery store if I chose to. When you search for it, you can find the good in things.

RELAXATION

Journaling, as mentioned above, represents one of many outlets for "passive recovery," a term that my colleague Dr. James Hoffmann has coined for ways that people can recover after rigorous training sessions. Of course, passive recovery can also apply to recovering from hard work and the extended periods of discipline that are needed to be successful in any endeavor. Additional examples of passive recovery tactics include the following: reading; watching television or a movie; listening to music; spending time with friends, family, and pets; playing a musical instrument; practicing some forms of yoga; or cooking and enjoying a good meal. (If you do choose to watch TV, don't get stuck in the habit of watching too much of it and putting off the other items listed in this chapter.) The key is that you allocate some time each day for you to unwind.

Those passive recovery techniques, as well as others that exist, can provide numerous health benefits. Among their many positive impacts, those activities can lower your heart rate and blood pressure; slow your breathing and decrease your metabolic stress; improve your overall mood; decrease anxiety; and lower perceived levels of fatigue.

The moral here is that periods of relaxation (in whatever form appeals most to you) are crucial if you want to be feeling your best and ready to tackle the next day's tasks. We cannot burn the candle from both ends; the more time that you can devote to relaxation (while still accomplishing all that you need to), the better off you will be. If you find it difficult to relax because you need to continue working toward success, remember that that's just your ego talking. You need to take time to relax and recharge. There are times, of course, when you need to push yourself harder than you ever have before, but those times must also be balanced by periods of relaxation and recovery. If you never let off the gas pedal, you'll eventually wear yourself out.

SLEEP

Movies and media suggest that those who are successful, especially at the highest level, work while others are sleeping. They're up at 4:00 a.m. and they're sleeping only a few hours each night. For most, that's not true. There is a fine line between working hard enough and long enough to accomplish your goals and also prioritizing yourself and taking care of yourself, which includes getting a proper amount of sleep. Not allowing your body to recharge impacts your mind, which also impacts your results—no matter the endeavor. As doctors James Hoffmann, Mike Israetel, and Melissa Davis outline in their book *Recovering from Training*, sleep is vital to success. "Sleep is a major regulator of autonomic balance," they write. "Sleep is thought to restore immunological and endocrine function, increase parasympathetic activity, and enhance memory consolidation, among other benefits. Larger amounts of growth hormone can also be released during sleep than during wakefulness, and this is thought to aid in tissue regeneration."

Even though sleep has been proven to offer all of these benefits, it's still overlooked by many people because they believe they are too busy. But being "too busy" most often means that you're not prioritizing the right things. And by not prioritizing the right tasks, you're working inefficiently, which limits the amount of time that you have to devote to everything else in your life. Inevitably, people are not prioritizing the time that they need for relaxation. The average person needs between 7 or 8 hours of sleep per night. But you also need to account for the time spent trying to fall asleep. If you stay disciplined and force yourself to go to bed at a reasonable time, you'll soon discover the difference that more sleep can make.

DAILY ROUTINES

Getting a head start on the day is generally beneficial, but there's no mandatory wake-up time that every successful person adheres to. It really is a personal preference. You have to figure out what works best for you, given your schedule and demands.

For me, I've found that I work best when I can be up a bit earlier than the rest of my family. It gives me time by myself when I can focus on my own needs before the needs of my family come into play. The same is true for social media. If I'm awake early enough—when not many other people are up and actively posting on Instagram, Facebook, or Twitter—there are fewer distractions that I have to deal with and I can better focus on what needs to get done.

Aristotle once said, "It is well to be up before daybreak, for such habits contribute to health, wealth, and wisdom." That premise is explored and substantiated by authors Robin Sharma (in *The 5 AM Club*) and Hal Elrod (in *The Miracle Morning*). If you develop a solid morning routine, for example, you can easily fit in exercise and reflection, as well as complete other important tasks, before other obligations in your life pull you in different directions.

Elrod outlines key principles or activities that make up a productive morning using the acronym SAVERS (Silence, Affirmations, Visualization, Exercise, Reading, and Scribing). Similarly, Sharma introduces a 20-20-20 plan, where a person devotes twenty minutes to exercise, twenty minutes to reflecting, and twenty minutes to education. Both are effective strategies for making sure those important activities and principles are incorporated into your morning routine. But it's important to note that these general principles can be applied to various lifestyles, including those in which early morning wake-ups are not the norm. The key is to set aside time for yourself each day—time to focus on improving yourself through exercise, through reflecting or meditation, and through a commitment to education. If you can calm your mind and better control your emotions, you'll be better at responding to external factors that are outside of your control.

Through these dedicated tasks you are also working on strengthening your personal willpower. It takes discipline to get up a bit earlier, to push yourself physically, and to focus on steadying your mind. If you can harness the benefits that come from these actions, you will continually improve. The differences may not be felt overnight, but marginal improvements that compound over weeks, months, and years can be powerful.

Here's how I structure my morning:

5:00 a.m. – Wake up and aim to do some type of cardio activity, such as rowing, running or incline walking on my treadmill.

5:30 a.m. – Create my to-do list for the day, make notes/journal, and examine my upcoming schedule.

6:00 a.m. – Shower and eat breakfast.

6:30 a.m. – Read at least fifty pages. (This takes thirty to sixty minutes to complete, depending on the complexity of the book and how many notes I am taking.)

7:30 a.m. – Be ready for my family to wake up, so I can help get their breakfast ready.

I typically go to bed around 10:00 at night. It takes discipline to try to get seven hours of sleep, but I have experimented with different times and routines, and I have found that when I commit to this particular schedule I typically feel my best. You may not experience immediate success by following this same routine, and that's okay. You must adjust it to fit your schedule. The main takeaway is to spend some time focusing on yourself and aiming to improve, at least a little bit, every single day.

You want to find a balance: working as hard as you need to without overdoing it. Pushing yourself and constantly making important decisions is draining. But if you can devote some time to focus on yourself—even if it seems next to impossible—you will emerge more productive. Remember, you must fix yourself before you can fix the world.

CONTINUED EDUCATION

As we covered earlier in this chapter, you can recharge by dedicating time to relaxation and activities that take your mind off of the tasks that occupy your time when you're in work mode. It can also be achieved by reading self-improvement books, which I experienced firsthand during the years that I spent learning how I could better myself as a person and business owner. (Incidentally, those years—and the hundreds of books read—became the research for *this* book.) As I saw for myself, the process of learning how you can improve yourself is a positive feedback loop. The more you learn and pick up new ideas from brilliant writers of the past and present, the more you can use those ideas to better yourself and your business.

You don't have to read a book a week or commit to anything too crazy, but you are likely missing out on opportunities to improve if you disregard the significance of reading books dedicated to bettering yourself. Even reading fiction can be beneficial—it can help lower stress levels and offer new perspectives.

Continued education doesn't only take the form of reading. It also includes listening to podcasts or attending seminars, either in person or online. Even keeping a daily journal can further your education, so long as you're keeping tabs on what you did well each day and what didn't go well. By chronicling those achievements and those setbacks—and by reviewing your journal with some regularity—you can learn how to be more successful in the future. All of these actions are investments in your future self, which offer incredible returns.

REAL WORLD VIEW

The principles outlined in this chapter may make sense or look good on paper, but if you're questioning how necessary they really are, consider that some of the most successful people in their fields implement them on a regular basis. Annie Thorisdottir, for example, prioritizes her diet and her sleep schedule. "The desire to be better is what drives me every day," she says, "and not eating right or getting enough sleep means not fully committing to becoming the best version of myself. I will not do that to myself. Proper nutrition and plenty of sleep is always a priority."

Similarly, Coach Bakich understands that he needs some downtime throughout the year, since recruiting and off-season training are a full-time commitment even before the season starts. "I take a few weeks off in the month of December for vacations and family time," he acknowledges. "That's a good recharge."

And even when she's on the road touring with her band, guitarist Nita Strauss still finds time for herself. "To me the best recharge is just a little simple self-care, taking a day or two to indulge in a little lazy time," she says. "Watch a show you like, sleep in, take a bath. The emails might pile up, but you'll escape burnout."

PUTTING IT INTO PRACTICE

Commit to bettering yourself by introducing new physical and mental activities into your daily and weekly routines. Whether you decide to start a comprehensive fitness regimen—or intensify an existing one—or you just begin walking a mile or two in the mornings or evenings during the week, this added (or new) exercise will not only improve your overall health, it will provide a nice balance to the strenuous work that occupies your typical work day. The same is true for your commitment to read more or to listen to educational podcasts.

CHAPTER 8

CONCLUSIONS

" —
People who succeed have momentum. The
more they succeed, the more they want
to succeed, and the more they find a
way to succeed."

—TONY ROBBINS

IF YOU WERE TO MAGICALLY OFFER a group of people six-pack abs or millions of dollars, I guarantee you that the vast majority of them would raise their hand to accept. But if you were to explain to that group of people what it takes to actually achieve washboard abs or to acquire millions of dollars, you'd be surprised how many people would lower their hands.

I've learned that people are always looking for a secret to success or a way to bypass a lot of the hard work. What I have discovered about the secret to success, however, is that there is no secret. Instead, it requires a relentless commitment to the basics. The sooner you learn and believe that, the faster you will achieve your own success (so long as you put in the hard work to get there). Take the quest for six-pack abs. Quick fixes, fads, and gimmicks won't get you there. The only thing that will is a commitment to work hard every single day for months, sometimes years. *That* is the secret to success.

The funny thing about success, especially in business, is that the people or companies that ultimately prove to be successful need a bit of momentum to get started. The fundamental principles outlined in this book can serve as your own boost of momentum. Once you achieve some preliminary success, it's important that you capitalize on it and use that as the driver to keep going. Putting in the time and the necessary effort won't be easy, but a long-term commitment is required if you want to maximize your potential success.

You're going to need to start with the foundation of a tenacious work ethic. Without it, the other principles outlined in this book won't amount to much. You can have the best ideas in the world, but without acting on them—in other words, without injecting them with a lot of hard work—they won't deliver success. Once you understand that hard work is paramount, you'll need to focus on what you can control. Sometimes you won't have the power to change the hand that you're dealt, but you can change how you respond to it. In doing so, you will empower yourself, and you'll learn the best course of action to overcome obstacles and to achieve success.

Throughout the entire process, a positive mindset and self-efficacy is crucial. This way of thinking, knowing that you can influence your outcomes via hard work, is what leads to personal growth. Whether you're an athlete or a businessperson, your mindset—and the actions that you take based on how you perceive the world around you—gives you the ability to influence outcomes. Assert your discipline to help you win the small, daily battles. Those will compound over the weeks, months, and years ahead. If you consistently create the right habits, you will slowly transform into a new (better) person.

You must also know your overall purpose. That will help you to push through the hard days when things go wrong and you find yourself questioning if all the hard work is really worth it. When your "why" is stronger than the struggle, you know you are on the right path. But make no mistake, you are going to struggle along the way. You will fail at times. Understanding this at the beginning and focusing on your sense of purpose will be your guide, keeping you on the right path to overcome these obstacles. You must also be prepared to learn from your mistakes. In doing so, you will grow and improve—and you'll be one step closer to success.

The fundamental nature of success's requisite hard work creates a dichotomy. It's easy to think that to be successful a person only needs to work hard. While hard work is absolutely necessary, being successful over the long term also requires a balance between work ethic and the willingness (and commitment) to recharge. You have to take proper care of your mind and your body if you want to maintain that necessary work ethic. And when you recharge, especially when you focus that time on self-improvement, you raise the ceiling of your potential success.

For my wife and me, cancer did not define our lives. It did not define our family. Instead, we changed our mindsets. We focused on being more optimistic, and we chose to focus only on the things that we could control. These were key factors that allowed us to get through Lori's battle with breast cancer, from the initial shock of the diagnosis through the surgical stage and the months of chemotherapy that followed. It would have been easy to play the victim card, especially when we, like much of the rest of the world, were forced to quarantine for months due to the coronavirus pandemic.

Yes, we were dealt a bad hand in 2020, but my wife and I refused to let it define us. Instead, we used the principles outlined in this book to make the most of it. The fundamental shift that we made in our mindset—to become more grateful for the little things and to focus on what we could control (instead of all of the uncertainty in the world)—allowed us to overcome the hardest battle that we had ever faced.

Success isn't relegated only to athletics or business careers. That lesson was made very clear to me in early 2020. Fortunately, the fundamental habits that are necessary for success in business or athletics are equally transferable to any facet of life. If you desire success, these are the principles that you must adopt and the habits that you must create. In doing so, you maximize your potential to achieve it.

RECOMMENDED READING

———

AS I WROTE THIS training guide for success, the following books provided inspiration. Several of them are referenced numerous times throughout the chapters, while others are only briefly mentioned. Regardless of the prominence of their role in this book, all are worth a read and all have contributed to my own success as a business owner, as well as my own personal growth as a husband, father, and coach.

13 Things Mentally Strong Parents Don't Do
Amy Morin

Adapt: Why Success Always Starts with Failure
Tim Harford

Being Wrong: Adventures in the Margin of Error
Kathryn Schulz

Built to Last: Successful Habits of Visionary Companies
Jim Collins and Jerry I. Porras

Choice or Chance: Understanding Your Locus of Control and Why It Matters
Stephen Nowicki

Recommended Reading

Delivering Happiness: A Path to Profits, Passion, and Purpose
Tony Hsieh

Drive: The Surprising Truth About What Motivates Us
Daniel H. Pink

Ego Is the Enemy
Ryan Holiday

Emotional Intelligence 2.0
Travis Bradberry and Jean Greaves

Endure: Mind, Body, and the Curiously Elastic Limits of Human Performance
Alex Hutchinson

Extreme Ownership: How U.S. Navy SEALs Lead and Win
Jocko Willink and Leif Babin

Find Your Why: A Practical Guide for Discovering Purpose for You and Your Team
Simon Sinek, David Mead, and Peter Docker

Flourish: A Visionary New Understanding of Happiness and Well-being
Martin E. P. Seligman

Flow: The Psychology of Optimal Experience
Mihaly Csikszentmihalyi

Genghis Khan and the Making of the Modern World
Jack Weatherford

Good to Great: Why Some Companies Make the Leap...and Others Don't
Jim Collins

Grit: The Power of Passion and Perseverance
Angela Duckworth

In Search of Excellence: Lessons from America's Best-Run Companies
Thomas J. Peters and Robert H. Waterman Jr.

Learned Optimism: How to Change Your Mind and Your Life
Martin E. P. Seligman

Legacy: What the All Blacks Can Teach Us About the Business of Life
James Kerr

Man's Search for Meaning
Viktor E. Frankl

Mindset: The New Psychology of Success
Carol S. Dweck

Nudge: Improving Decisions about Health, Wealth, and Happiness

Recommended Reading

Richard H. Thaler and Cass R. Sunstein
Outliers: The Story of Success
Malcolm Gladwell

Peak: Secrets from the New Science of Expertise
Anders Ericsson and Robert Pool

Range: Why Generalists Triumph in a Specialized World
David Epstein

Recovering from Training: How to Manage Fatigue to Maximize Performance
James Hoffmann, Mike Israetel, and Melissa Davis

Relentless: From Good to Great to Unstoppable
Tim S. Grover

Shoe Dog: A Memoir by the Creator of Nike
Phil Knight

Stumbling on Happiness
Daniel Gilbert

The 5AM Club: Own Your Morning. Elevate Your Life.
Robin Sharma

The 7 Habits of Highly Effective People: Powerful Lessons in Personal Change
Stephen R. Covey

The Impulse Society: America in the Age of Instant Gratification
Paul Roberts

The Lean Startup: How Today's Entrepreneurs Use Continuous Innovation to Create Radically Successful Businesses
Eric Ries

The Millionaire Next Door: The Surprising Secrets of America's Wealthy
Thomas J. Stanley and William D. Danko

The Miracle Morning: The Not-So-Obvious Secret Guaranteed to Transform Your Life (Before 8AM)
Hal Elrod

The Obstacle Is the Way: The Timeless Art of Turning Trials into Triumph
Ryan Holiday

The Power of Habit: Why We Do What We Do in Life and Business
Charles Duhigg

The Renaissance Diet 2.0
Mike Israetel, Melissa Davis, Jen Case, and James Hoffmann

The Richest Man in Babylon
George S. Clason

Recommended Reading

The Sports Gene: Inside the Science of Extraordinary Athletic Performance
David Epstein

The Success Equation: Untangling Skill and Luck in Business, Sports, and Investing
Michael J. Mauboussin

The Warrior Elite: The Forging of SEAL Class 228
Dick Couch

The Willpower Instinct: How Self-Control Works, Why It Matters, and What You Can Do to Get More of It
Kelly McGonigal

Think and Grow Rich
Napoleon Hill

Thinking, Fast and Slow
Daniel Kahneman

Understanding Healthy Eating: A Science-Based Guide to How Your Diet Affects Your Health
Mike Israetel, Jen Case, and Trevor Pfaendtner

Why Smart Executives Fail: And What You Can Learn from Their Mistakes
Sydney Finkelstein

Willpower: Rediscovering the Greatest Human Strength
Roy F. Baumeister and John Tierney

ACKNOWLEDGMENTS

—

I MUST BEGIN BY thanking my wife, Lori Shaw, for inspiring me to write this book. Even as she battled through breast cancer this year, she always put her family first. Her strength—both physical and emotional—as well as her mindset and her character continue to fill me with awe. Thank you, Lori, for your unwavering support in my journey to build a successful fitness company and to write this book.

I also must express sincere gratitude to my parents, who raised me to value hard work and to understand the importance of doing the right thing. They have always encouraged and supported me in the pursuit of my dreams, whether those aspirations were academic, athletic, or business-focused.

I consider myself to be incredibly fortunate. I have met and worked alongside a number of impressive individuals. My biggest mentor, Dr. Mike Israetel, is also one of my best friends and the co-founder of Renaissance Periodization (RP). He has constantly challenged me to reevaluate how I think, and he has been instrumental in developing my approach to fitness, work, and life. Without his help and guidance, Renaissance Periodization—and likely this book—would not exist.

Acknowledgements

They say that if you are the smartest person in the room, then you are in the wrong room. Luckily for me, that has never been the case. I have been constantly surrounded by some of the best and the brightest individuals in the fitness industry. To all of the RP coaches, employees, and contractors: thank you for making Renaissance Periodization what it is today. I couldn't do it without you. And thank you to the app engineering team for making the RP methodology accessible to the masses.

A special thanks to Shaun Tolson, whose expertise and help editing this book was instrumental to its success. Also, thanks to my colleague Tiago Faleiro for his feedback and insight after reading early drafts of every chapter.

Get in the best shape of your life with the RP Diet App, designed to be your personal diet coach in your pocket and all for less than $15/month. The RP Diet App helps create a custom diet for you based on your schedule, lifestyle, and goals. It updates weekly based on your progress. The RP Diet App has helped tens of thousands of individuals around the world reach their health and fitness goals. Download the app in the Apple and/or Google Play stores to get started today!

MEET YOUR NEW DIET COACH

Start your transformation today with your free 14-day trial.

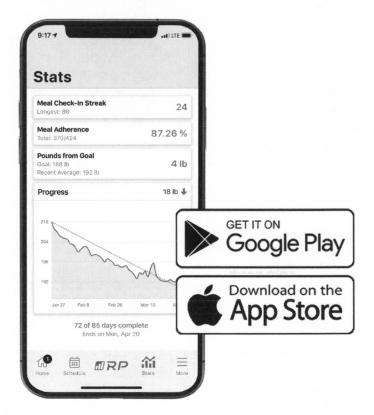

INDEX

___